Length Tension Testing Book 2, Upper Quadrant

Length Tension Testing Book 2, Upper Quadrant

A WORKBOOK OF MANUAL THERAPY TECHNIQUES

SECOND EDITION

Paolo Sanzo, DScPT, MSc, BScPT, FCAMT
Murray MacHutchon, BMRPT, FCAMT

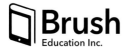

Brush Education Inc.

Brush Education Inc.
www.brusheducation.ca
contact@brusheducation.ca

Photographer: Allan Dickson Photography
Model: Melinda Vaillant
Cover design: Dean Pickup
Interior design: Carol Dragich, Dragich Design

Printed and manufactured in Canada

Library and Archives Canada Cataloguing in Publication
Sanzo, Paolo, 1969–, author
Length tension testing : a workbook of manual therapy techniques /
Paolo Sanzo, DScPT, MSC, BSCPT, FCAMT, Murray MacHutchon,
BMRPT, FCAMT. — Second edition.

Originally published in 2007. Includes bibliographical references.
Contents: Book 1. Lower quadrant — Book 2. Upper quadrant. Issued in
print and electronic formats. ISBN 978-1-55059-596-3 (pbk. : bk. 2).—
ISBN 978-1-55059-594-9 (mobi : bk. 1).— ISBN 978-1-55059-597-0
(pdf : bk. 2).— ISBN 978-1-55059-599-4 (epub : bk. 2)

1. Physical therapy.   I. MacHutchon, Murray, author   II. Title.

RM700.S36 2015   615.8′2   C2014-907343-7
                                         C2014-907344-5

We acknowledge the financial support of the Government of Canada
through the Canada Book Fund for our publishing activities.

Acknowledgements

Together we are thankful for all the dedicated and hard working physiotherapists who have volunteered countless hours to make the Orthopaedic Division of the Canadian Physiotherapy Association a success and recognized all over the world.

We are also thankful to our ever-loving families who are supportive in all of our endeavors.

Contents

Introduction

Assessment

The assessment of length tension in muscle involves the use of clinical reasoning and interpretation of the subjective and objective assessment findings. These findings include:

- the referral pattern of pain;
- positional findings on observation;
- changes in active and passive range of motion;
- findings on palpation; and
- activation of the muscle and the flexibility of the muscle during the length tension assessment of the myofascial structures.

Differentiation must also be made in the tension and barrier that are palpated in order to determine whether this is due to the myofascial tissue or the neuromeningeal tissue. Conclusions are then based on these combined tests and the muscle is determined to be normal, hypertonic, shortened or lengthened.

The therapist may incorporate principles of neuromeningeal assessment in order to assess whether the tension and barrier present is due to the myofascial tissues or due to the neuromeningeal structures. Excellent resources are available on the assessment of neuromeningeal tissue, and readers are advised to refer to these for further information and more details. Therapists must have an appreciation for the uniqueness of our anatomy. All tension testing described in this book may have to be slightly altered to accommodate the examiner's or the patient's anatomy.

End feel

The different sensations imparted to the hand of the therapist at the extremes of the passive range of motion is termed the *end feel*. The end feel caused by changes in the myofascial system will be different from some of the end feels associated with a joint restriction.

Normal muscle at rest, and preferably with gravity eliminated, will feel soft. It will have the same feel as palpating raw steak or soft tofu. The length and tension will be as expected for the age of the patient. The contralateral muscle can be tested to confirm this. A normal muscle will contract with voluntary electromyographic (EMG) activity.

Hypertonic muscle has increased elastic and viscoelastic stiffness in the absence of contractile activity. Palpation of the hypertonic muscle will feel similar to palpating well done steak and it will have decreased length on testing. Muscle spasm is an abnormal muscle contraction and is often painful. The EMG activity is not under voluntary control. This strong contraction will limit movement significantly. A muscle spasm is velocity dependent. If the muscle is lengthened or moved quickly, an increase in muscle tone is evident.

Truly shortened muscle, or a muscle contracture, is often present post trauma and will feel gristly, tight and short on testing. The muscle contractile unit is shortened in the absence of EMG activity. When the muscle is lengthened or moved, the response is velocity independent. It does not matter if the movement is performed quickly or slowly, the response and length remains unchanged.

The therapist must recognize the different sensations imparted to the hands at the end of the available passive range of motion and gently sense the point at which the range of motion stops. It is with our palpation skills that we determine that it is in fact the muscle being tested that is felt to be tense and that is providing the resistance to the passive movement. Both the hand providing stabilization and the hand moving the body part must together sense the tension in the muscle and the barrier present.

Clinical reasoning

Length tension test findings may be unrelated to the palpation findings found in muscle at rest. As previously explained, the therapist must base their conclusions on a clinical reasoning approach to rule out other problems or tissues at fault. Length tension testing should preferably be performed in supine lying or prone lying to unload the muscle and neutralize the effect of gravity. This cannot always be done, however, and thus alternative test positions are also described.

Disclaimer

The procedures described in this book should be implemented in a manner consistent with professional standards set for the circumstances that apply in each situation. Every effort has been made to confirm accuracy of the information presented and to correctly relate generally accepted practices.

Nevertheless, practitioners must always rely on their own experience, knowledge, and judgment when consulting any of the information contained in this reference or employing it in patient care. When using any of this information, they should remain conscious of their responsibility for their own safety and the safety of others, and for the best interests of those in their care.

To the fullest extent of the law, neither the publishers, the authors, nor the editors assume any liability for injury or damage to persons or property from any use of information or ideas contained in this reference.

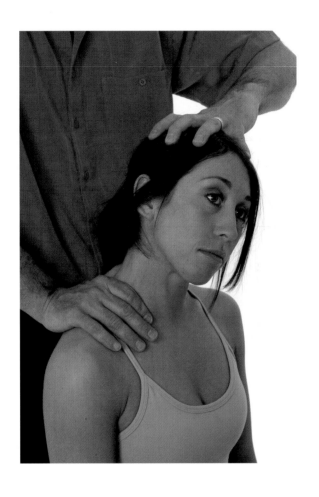

Trapezius—Upper Fibers

Technique 1

Technique described for the right trapezius muscle.

Patient: Positioned in supine lying with the arms resting by the side and the knees flexed.

Therapist: Standing at the head of the bed.

Action: Support the posterior aspect of the patient's head with both hands and then passively flex the craniovertebral joint. Your right hand stabilizes the lateral one-third of the patient's right clavicle and acromion while palpating the muscle. Using your left hand, gently and slowly flex, left-side flex and right rotate the mid and lower cervical spine. Both the stabilizing hand and the hand moving the body part sense the tension in the muscle and barrier. Assess the amount of range and the end feel and note the reproduction of any symptoms. Repeat this test on the contralateral side and compare the two results.

Note also the reproduction of any dural symptoms. To differentiate between neuromeningeal tissue and the patient's muscle, add various sensitizing movements of the upper extremities and note any change in the amount of range, the end feel and the symptoms produced.

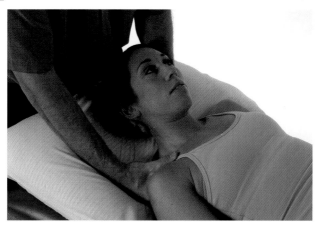

Trapezius—Upper Fibers

Technique 2
Technique described for the right trapezius muscle.

Patient: Positioned in sitting.

Therapist: Standing behind the patient.

Action: The patient actively flexes their craniovertebral joint. Use your right hand to stabilize the lateral one-third of the patient's right clavicle and acromion while palpating the muscle. Using your left hand, passively flex, left-side flex and right rotate the mid and lower cervical spine. Both the stabilizing hand and the hand moving the body part sense the tension in the muscle and barrier. Assess the amount of range and the end feel and note the reproduction of any symptoms. Repeat this test on the contralateral side and compare the two results.

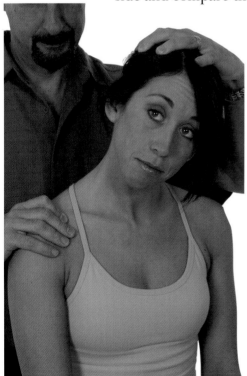

Note also the reproduction of any dural symptoms. To differentiate between neuromeningeal tissue and the patient's muscle, add various sensitizing movements of the upper extremities and note any change in the amount of range, the end feel and the symptoms produced.

Trapezius—Middle Fibers

Technique 1
Technique described for the right trapezius muscle.

Patient: Positioned in prone lying with the arms resting by their side and the neck resting in right rotation.

Therapist: Standing on the left side of the bed.

Action: Stabilize the left transverse processes of T1 to T5 with the palmar aspect of your left hand. Employing a cross-hand technique, use your right hand to depress and protract the lateral aspect of the patient's right scapula. Both the stabilizing hand and the hand moving the body part sense the tension in the muscle and barrier. Assess the amount of range and the end feel and note the reproduction of any symptoms. Repeat this test on the contralateral side and compare the two results.

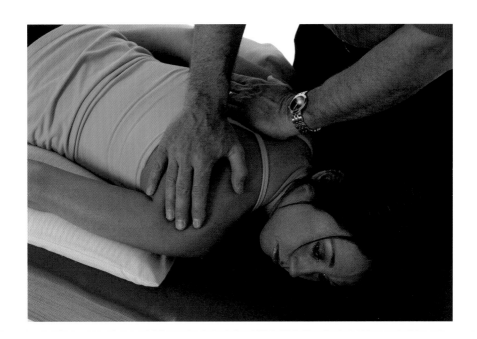

Trapezius—Middle Fibers

Technique 2
Technique described for the right trapezius muscle.

Patient: Positioned in left side lying with a pillow
between the knees.

Therapist: Standing on the left side of the bed, facing
the patient.

Action: Grasp the inferior aspect of the medial and
lateral border of the patient's right scapula with your
left hand and the superior aspect of the medial and
lateral border of their right scapula with your right
hand. Depress and protract the patient's right scapula. Both the stabilizing hand and the hand moving
the body part sense the tension in the muscle and
barrier. Assess the amount of range and the end feel
and note the reproduction of any symptoms. Repeat
this test on the contralateral side and compare the
two results.

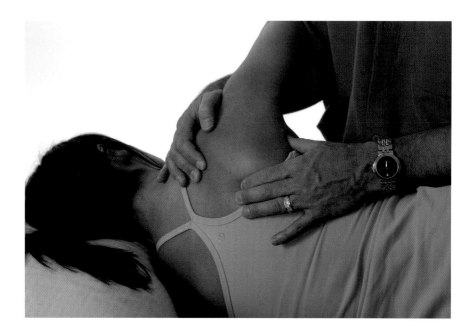

Trapezius—Lower Fibers

Technique 1
Technique described for the right trapezius muscle.

Patient: Positioned in prone lying with the arms resting by their side and the neck resting in right rotation.

Therapist: Standing on the left side of the bed.

Action: Stabilize the left transverse processes of T6 to T12 with the palmar aspect of your left hand. Employing a cross-hand technique, use your right hand to elevate, protract and downwardly rotate the patient's right scapula so that the glenoid faces inferiorly. Both the stabilizing hand and the hand moving the body part sense the tension in the muscle and barrier. Assess the amount of range and the end feel and note the reproduction of any symptoms. Repeat this test on the contralateral side and compare the two results.

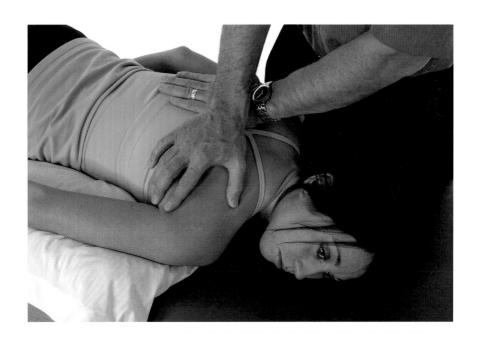

Trapezius—Lower Fibers

Technique 2
Technique described for the right trapezius muscle.

Patient: Positioned in left side lying with a pillow between the knees.

Therapist: Standing on the left side of the bed, facing the patient.

Action: Grasp the inferior aspect of the medial and lateral border of the patient's right scapula with your left hand and the superior aspect of the medial and lateral border of their right scapula with your right hand. Elevate, protract and downwardly rotate the patient's right scapula so that the glenoid faces inferiorly. Both the stabilizing hand and the hand moving the body part sense the tension in the muscle and barrier. Assess the amount of range and the end feel and note the reproduction of any symptoms. Repeat this test on the contralateral side and compare the two results.

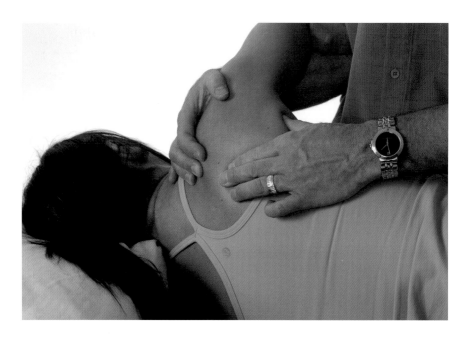

Rectus Capitis Posterior Major

Technique 1
Technique described for the right rectus capitis posterior major muscle.

Patient: Positioned in supine lying with the knees flexed.

Therapist: Standing at the head of the bed.

Action: Grasp and stabilize the axis using the web space of your left hand. With your right hand, grasp the inferior aspect of the occiput in a football hold, resting your anterior shoulder against the patient's forehead. Flex and rotate the occiput to the left. Both the stabilizing hand and the hand moving the body part sense the tension in the muscle and barrier. Assess the amount of range and the end feel and note the reproduction of any symptoms. Repeat this test on the contralateral side and compare the two results.

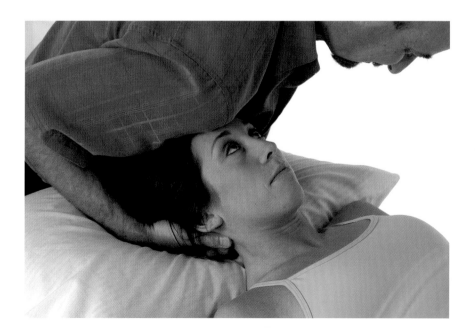

Rectus Capitis Posterior Major

Technique 2
Technique described for the right rectus capitis posterior major muscle.

Patient: Positioned in sitting.

Therapist: Standing on the left side of the patient.

Action: Grasp and stabilize the axis using the web space of your right hand. With your left hand, grasp the inferior aspect of the patient's occiput in a football hold, with the ulnar border of your left 5th digit cupped under the inferior aspect of the occiput. Support the anterior aspect of the patient's forehead with your left biceps and forearm. Flex and rotate the occiput to the left. Both the stabilizing hand and the hand moving the body part sense the tension in the muscle and barrier. Assess the amount of range and the end feel and note the reproduction of any symptoms. Repeat this test on the contralateral side and compare the two results.

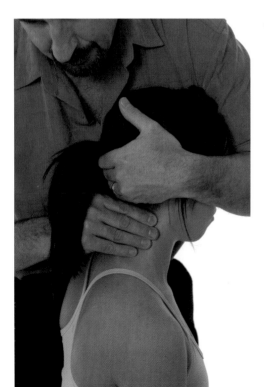

Rectus Capitis Posterior Minor

Technique 1

Technique described for the right rectus capitis posterior minor muscle.

Patient: Positioned in supine lying with the knees flexed.

Therapist: Standing at the head of the bed.

Action: Grasp and stabilize the atlas using the web space of your left hand. With your right hand, grasp the inferior aspect of the occiput in a football hold, resting your anterior shoulder against the patient's forehead. Flex the occiput. Both the stabilizing hand and the hand moving the body part sense the tension in the muscle and barrier. Assess the amount of range and the end feel and note the reproduction of any symptoms. Repeat this test on the contralateral side and compare the two results.

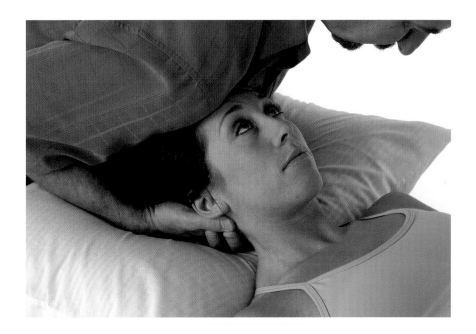

Rectus Capitis Posterior Minor

Technique 2
Technique described for the right rectus capitis
posterior minor muscle.

Patient: Positioned in sitting.

Therapist: Standing on the left side of the patient.

Action: Grasp and stabilize the atlas using the web
space of your right hand. With your left hand, grasp
the inferior aspect of the patient's occiput in a football hold, with the ulnar border of your left 5th digit
cupped under the inferior aspect of the occiput.
Support the anterior aspect of the patient's forehead
with your biceps and forearm. Flex the occiput. Both
the stabilizing hand and the hand moving the body
part sense the tension in the muscle and barrier.
Assess the amount of range
and the end feel and
note the reproduction
of any symptoms.
Repeat this test on
the contralateral side
and compare the two
results.

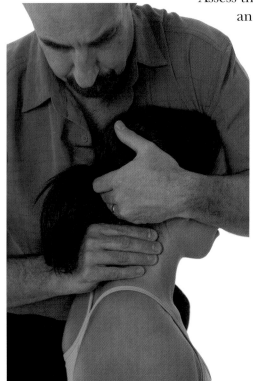

Superior Oblique

Technique 1
Technique described for the right superior oblique muscle.

Patient: Positioned in supine lying with the knees flexed.

Therapist: Standing at the head of the bed.

Action: Grasp and stabilize the atlas using the web space of your left hand. With your right hand, grasp the inferior aspect of the occiput in a football hold, resting your anterior shoulder against the patient's forehead. Flex and side-flex the occiput to the left. Both the stabilizing hand and the hand moving the body part sense the tension in the muscle and barrier. Assess the amount of range and the end feel and note the reproduction of any symptoms. Repeat this test on the contralateral side and compare the two results.

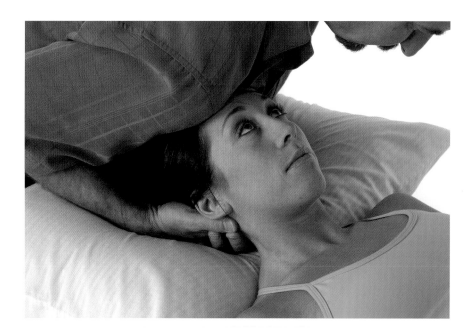

Superior Oblique

Technique 2

Technique described for the right superior oblique
muscle.

Patient: Positioned in sitting.

Therapist: Standing to the left of the patient.

Action: Grasp and stabilize the atlas using the web
space of your right hand. With your left hand, grasp
the inferior aspect of the occiput in a football hold,
with the ulnar border of your left 5th digit cupped
under the inferior aspect of the occiput. Support the
anterior aspect of the patient's forehead with your
biceps and forearm. Flex and side flex the occiput
to the left. Both the stabilizing hand and the hand
moving the body part sense the tension in the muscle
and barrier. Assess the amount of range and the end
feel and note the reproduction of any symptoms.
Repeat this test on the contra-
lateral side and compare the
two results.

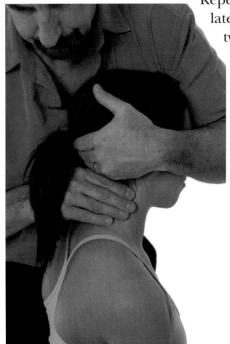

Inferior Oblique

Technique 1

Technique described for the right inferior oblique muscle.

Patient: Positioned in supine lying with the knees flexed.

Therapist: Standing at the head of the bed.

Action: Grasp and stabilize the axis using the web space of your left hand. Using the web space of your right hand, grasp the inferior aspect of the atlas, resting your anterior shoulder against the patient's forehead. Rotate and side-flex the atlas to the left. Both the stabilizing hand and the hand moving the body part sense the tension in the muscle and barrier. Assess the amount of range and the end feel and note the reproduction of any symptoms. Repeat this test on the contralateral side and compare the two results.

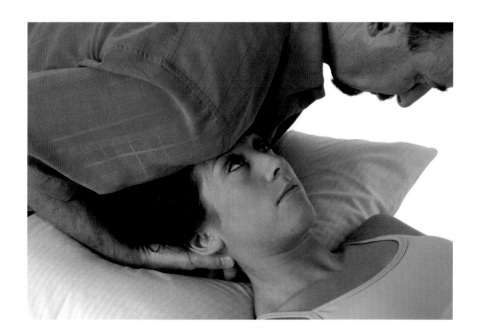

Inferior Oblique

Technique 2
Technique described for the right inferior oblique muscle.

Patient: Positioned in sitting.

Therapist: Standing to the left of the patient.

Action: Grasp and stabilize the axis using the web space of your right hand. With your left hand, grasp the inferior aspect of the atlas in a football hold, with the ulnar border of your left 5th digit cupped under the inferior aspect of the atlas. Support the anterior aspect of the patient's forehead with your biceps and forearm. Rotate and side-flex the atlas to the left. Both the stabilizing hand and the hand moving the body part sense the tension in the muscle and barrier. Assess the amount of range and the end feel and note the reproduction of any symptoms. Repeat this test on the contralateral side and compare the two results.

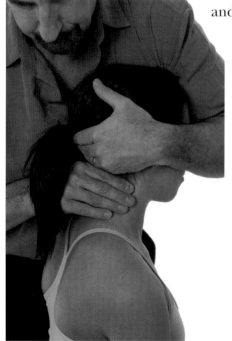

Scalene Anterior

Technique 1
Technique described for the right scalene anterior
muscle.

Patient: Positioned in supine lying with the knees flexed.

Therapist: Standing at the head of the bed.

Action: Support the patient's cervical spine and occiput
with your left hand while stabilizing their 1st rib
with your right hand. The patient's cervical spine is
extended, side-flexed to the left and rotated to the
right. Both the stabilizing hand and the hand moving
the body part sense the tension in the muscle and
barrier. Assess the amount of range and the end feel
and note the reproduction of any symptoms. Repeat
this test on the contralateral side and compare the
two results.

(Technique continued on next page.)

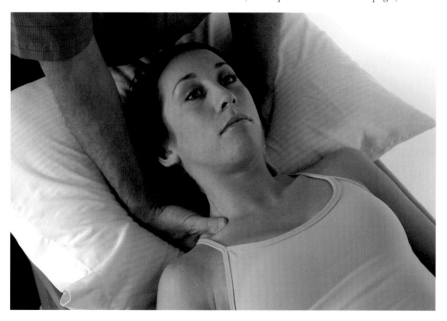

Note also the reproduction of any dural symptoms.
To differentiate between neuromeningeal tissue
and the patient's muscle, add various sensitizing
movements of the upper extremities and note any
change in the amount of range, the end feel and the
symptoms produced.

Scalene Anterior

Technique 2
Technique described for the right scalene anterior muscle.

Patient: Positioned in sitting.

Therapist: Standing behind the patient or to the left of the patient.

Action: With your right hand, stabilize and palpate the attachment of the muscle on the 1st rib. Place your left hand on the superior aspect of the patient's occiput and extend the cervical spine. You may also use a football grip to position the patient's cervical spine into extension. The cervical spine is then side-flexed to the left and rotated to the right. Both the stabilizing hand and the hand moving the body part sense the tension in the muscle and barrier. Assess the amount of range and the end feel and note the reproduction of any symptoms. Repeat this test on the contralateral side and compare the two results.

Note also the reproduction of any dural symptoms. To differentiate between neuromeningeal tissue and the patient's muscle, add various sensitizing movements of the upper extremities and note any change in the amount of range, the end feel and the symptoms produced.

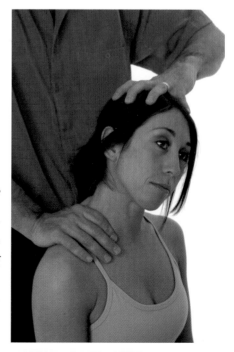

Scalene Medius

Technique 1

Technique described for the right scalene medius muscle.

Patient: Positioned in supine lying with the knees flexed.

Therapist: Standing at the head of the bed.

Action: With your right hand, stabilize and palpate the attachment of the muscle on the 1st rib, with your left hand supporting the cervical spine and occiput in neutral flexion and extension. The patient's cervical spine is then side-flexed to the left and rotated to the right side. Both the stabilizing hand and the hand moving the body part sense the tension in the muscle and barrier. Assess the amount of range and the end feel and note the reproduction of any symptoms. Repeat this test on the contralateral side and compare the two results.

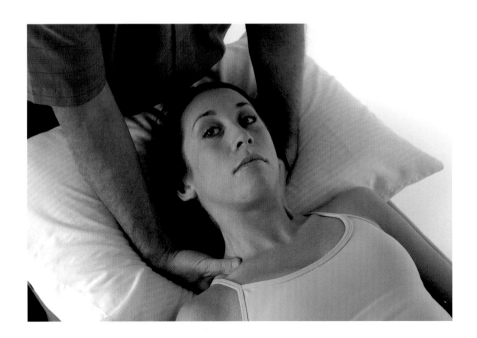

Note also the reproduction of any dural symptoms.
To differentiate between neuromeningeal tissue
and the patient's muscle, add various sensitizing
movements of the upper extremities and note any
change in the amount of range, the end feel and the
symptoms produced.

Scalene Medius

Technique 2

Technique described for the right scalene medius
muscle.

Patient: Positioned in sitting.

Therapist: Standing behind or to the left of the patient.

Action: With your right hand, palpate and stabilize the
attachment of the muscle on the 1st rib. Place your
left hand on the superior aspect of the patient's
occiput and keep the cervical spine in neutral flexion and extension. Alternatively, you can accomplish
this by using a football grip instead. The cervical
spine is then side-flexed to the left and rotated to the
right. Both the stabilizing hand and the hand moving
the body part sense the tension in the muscle and
barrier. Assess the amount of range and the end feel
and note the reproduction of any symptoms. Repeat
this test on the contralateral side and compare the
two results.

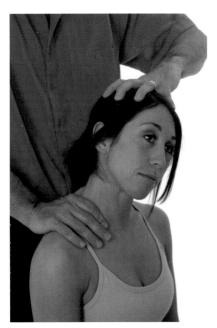

Note also the repro-
duction of any dural
symptoms. To dif-
ferentiate between
neuromeningeal tissue
and the patient's muscle,
add various sensitizing
movements of the upper
extremities and note any
change in the amount of
range, the end feel and
the symptoms produced.

Scalene Posterior

Technique 1
Technique described for the right scalene posterior muscle.

Patient: Positioned in supine lying with the knees flexed.

Therapist: Standing at the head of the bed.

Action: With your right hand, palpate and stabilize the attachment of the muscle on the 2nd rib while supporting the patient's cervical spine and occiput with your left hand. The patient's cervical spine is flexed and side-flexed and rotated to the left. Then ask the patient to expire, and with your right hand apply an inferior glide to the 2nd rib. Both the stabilizing hand and the hand moving the body part sense the tension in the muscle and barrier. Assess the amount of range and the end feel and note the reproduction of any symptoms. Repeat this test on the contralateral side and compare the two results.

(Technique continued on next page.)

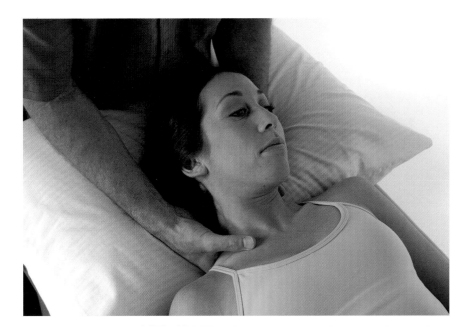

Note also the reproduction of any dural symptoms.
To differentiate between neuromeningeal tissue
and the patient's muscle, add various sensitizing
movements of the upper extremities and note any
change in the amount of range, the end feel and the
symptoms produced.

Scalene Posterior

Technique 2

Technique described for the right scalene posterior muscle.

Patient: Positioned in sitting.

Therapist: Standing behind the patient.

Action: Place your left hand on the superior aspect of the patient's occiput and flex their cervical spine. Alternatively, you can accomplish this flexion by using a football grip instead. The cervical spine is then side-flexed and rotated to the left side. Ask the patient to expire and with your right hand apply an inferior glide to the 2nd rib. Both the stabilizing hand and the hand moving the body part sense the tension in the muscle and barrier. Assess the amount of range and the end feel and note the reproduction of any symptoms. Repeat this test on the contralateral side and compare the two results.

Note also the reproduction of any dural symptoms. To differentiate between neuromeningeal tissue and the patient's muscle, add various sensitizing movements of the upper extremities and note any change in the amount of range, the end feel and the symptoms produced.

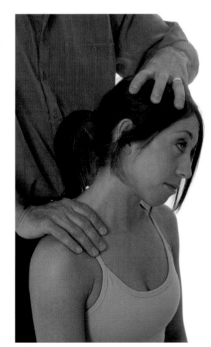

Sternocleidomastoid

Technique 1
Technique described for the right sternocleidomastoid muscle.

Patient: Positioned in supine lying with the knees flexed.

Therapist: Standing at the head of the bed.

Action: With your right hand, stabilize and palpate the attachment of the muscle on the medial one-third of the right clavicle as you gently take up the tension. Supporting the patient's cervical spine and occiput with your left hand, the patient's craniovertebral joint is flexed and the cervical spine is extended, side-flexed to the left and rotated to the right. Both the stabilizing hand and the hand moving the body part sense the tension in the muscle and barrier. Assess the amount of range and the end feel and note the reproduction of any symptoms. Repeat this test on the contralateral side and compare the two results.

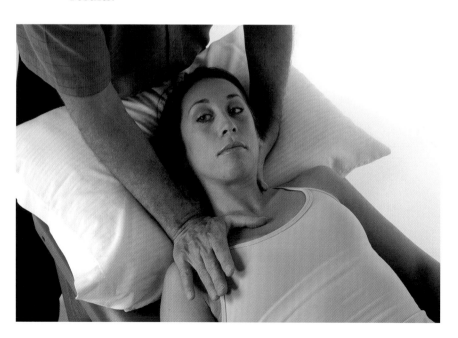

Note also the reproduction of any dural symptoms. To differentiate between neuromeningeal tissue and the patient's muscle, add various sensitizing movements of the upper extremities and note any change in the amount of range, the end feel and the symptoms produced.

Sternocleidomastoid

Technique 2
Technique described for the right sternocleidomastoid
muscle.

Patient: Positioned in sitting.

Therapist: Standing behind the patient.

Action: With your right hand, stabilize and palpate the
attachment of the muscle on the medial one-third of
the right clavicle as you gently take up the tension.
Ask the patient to flex their craniovertebral joint and
maintain this position. Then, placing your left hand
on the superior aspect of the patient's occiput, the
cervical spine is extended, side-flexed to the left and
rotated to the right. Both the stabilizing hand and
the hand moving the body part sense the tension in
the muscle and barrier. Assess the amount of range
and the end feel and note the reproduction of any
symptoms. Repeat this test on the contralateral side
and compare the two results.

Note also the reproduction of any dural
symptoms. To differentiate between neuromeningeal tissue and the patient's
muscle, add various sensitizing
movements of the upper
extremities and note any
change in the amount of
range, the end feel and the
symptoms produced.

Levator Scapulae

Technique 1

Technique described for the right levator scapulae muscle.

Patient: Positioned in supine lying with the knees flexed.

Therapist: Standing at the head of the bed.

Action: Using your right hand, stabilize the superior and medial border of the right scapula and palpate the attachment of the muscle. Supporting the patient's cervical spine and occiput with your left hand, the cervical spine is then flexed, side-flexed and rotated to the left, while depressing the right scapula with your right hand. Both the stabilizing hand and the hand moving the body part sense the tension in the muscle and barrier. Assess the amount of range and the end feel and note the reproduction of any symptoms. Repeat this test on the contralateral side and compare the two results.

(Technique continued on next page.)

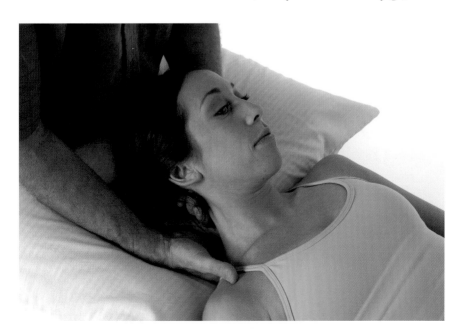

You may also ask the patient to actively abduct their right shoulder overhead and flex their right elbow. This position allows their right scapula to rotate upward so that the glenoid is facing superiorly, adding further tension to the muscle. Both the stabilizing hand and the hand moving the body part sense the tension in the muscle and barrier. Assess the amount of range and the end feel and note the reproduction of any symptoms. Repeat this test on the contralateral side and compare the two results.

Levator Scapulae

Technique 2
Technique described for the right levator scapulae muscle.

Patient: Positioned in sitting.

Therapist: Standing behind the patient.

Action: Stabilize the superior and medial border of the right scapula and palpate the attachment of the muscle with your right hand. Support the patient's cervical spine and occiput with your left hand. The cervical spine is then flexed, side-flexed and rotated to the left, also with your left hand. Both the stabilizing hand and the hand moving the body part sense the tension in the muscle and barrier. Assess the amount of range and the end feel and note the reproduction of any symptoms. Repeat this test on the contralateral side and compare the two results.

You may also ask the patient to actively abduct their right shoulder overhead and flex their right elbow. This position allows their right scapula to rotate upward so that the glenoid is facing superiorly, adding further tension to the muscle. Both the stabilizing hand and the hand moving the body part sense the tension in the muscle and barrier. Assess the amount of range and the end feel and note the reproduction of any symptoms. Repeat this test on the contralateral side and compare the two results.

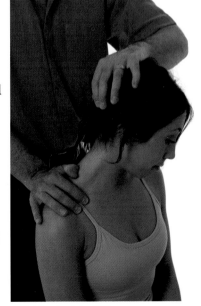

Splenius Capitis

Technique 1

Technique described for the right splenius capitis muscle.

Patient: Positioned in supine lying with the knees flexed.

Therapist: Standing at the head of the bed.

Action: Stabilize the spinous processes from C7 to T3 with your left hand. Ask the patient to actively flex their craniovertebral joint and maintain this position. Then, supporting the cervical spine and occiput with your right hand, the cervical spine is flexed, left side-flexed and left rotated. Both the stabilizing hand and the hand moving the body part sense the tension in the muscle and barrier. Assess the amount of range and the end feel and note the reproduction of any symptoms. Repeat this test on the contralateral side and compare the two results.

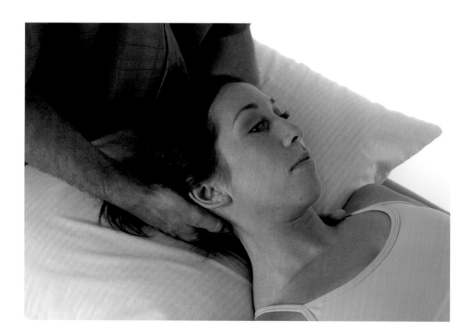

Splenius Capitis

Technique 2

Technique described for the right splenius capitis muscle.

Patient: Positioned in sitting.

Therapist: Standing behind the patient.

Action: Stabilize the spinous processes from C7 to T3 with your right hand. Ask the patient to actively flex their craniovertebral joint and maintain this position. You then support the patient's cervical spine and occiput with your left hand. Alternatively, you can accomplish this flexion by using a football grip. The patient's cervical spine is then flexed, left side-flexed and left rotated. Both the stabilizing hand and the hand moving the body part sense the tension in the muscle and barrier. Assess the amount of range and the end feel and note the reproduction of any symptoms. Repeat this test on the contralateral side and compare the two results.

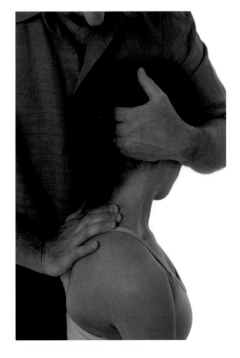

Splenius Cervicis

Technique 1
Technique described for the right splenius cervicis
muscle.

Patient: Positioned in supine lying with the knees flexed.

Therapist: Standing at the head of the bed.

Action: Stabilize the spinous processes from T3 to T6
with your left hand. Supporting the patient's upper
cervical spine from C1 to C4 with your right hand,
the upper cervical spine is then flexed, side-flexed
and rotated to the left. Both the stabilizing hand and
the hand moving the body part sense the tension in
the muscle and barrier. Assess the amount of range
and the end feel and note the reproduction of any
symptoms. Repeat this test on the contralateral side
and compare the two results.

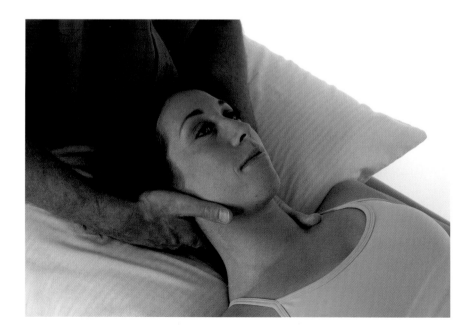

Splenius Cervicis

Technique 2

Technique described for the right splenius cervicis
muscle.

Patient: Positioned in sitting.

Therapist: Standing to the left side of the patient.

Action: Stabilize the spinous processes from T3 to T6
   with your right hand. Then support the patient's
   upper cervical spine from C1 to C4 with your left
   hand, using a football hold, with the anterior aspect
   of the patient's forehead supported by your left
   biceps and forearm. The patient's upper cervical
   spine from C1 to C4 is then flexed and side-flexed
   and rotated to the left. Both the stabilizing hand and
   the hand moving the body part sense the tension in
   the muscle and barrier. Assess the amount of range
   and the end feel and note the reproduction of any
   symptoms. Repeat this
   test on the contralateral
   side and compare the
   two results.

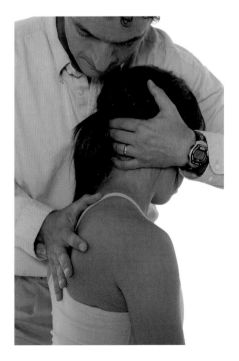

THE TEMPOROMANDIBULAR JOINT

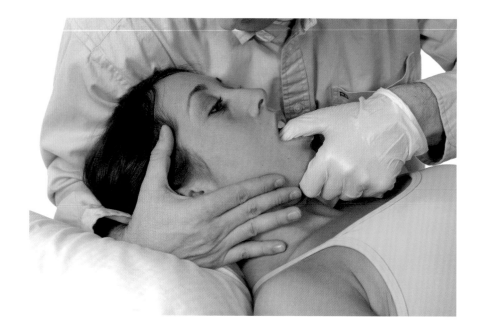

Medial Pterygoid

Technique 1

Technique described for the right medial pterygoid muscle.

Patient: Positioned in supine lying with the knees flexed.

Therapist: Standing on the left side of the bed with a non-latex glove on the left hand.

Action: Support and stabilize the patient's occiput with your right hand using a football hold, cradling the posterior aspect of the occiput with your right biceps and forearm. Place your left thumb along the patient's molars and your left index finger on the inferior aspect of the mandible. Then use your left hand to open, retrude and laterally glide the mandible to the right. Both the stabilizing hand and the hand moving the body part sense the tension in the muscle and barrier. Assess the amount of range and the end feel and note the reproduction of any symptoms. Repeat this test on the contralateral side and compare the two results.

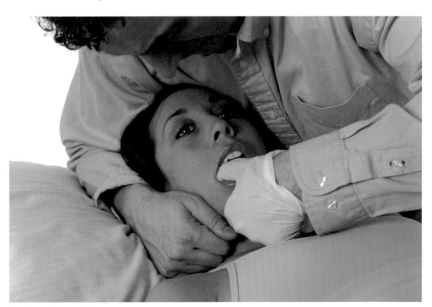

Medial Pterygoid

Technique 2
Technique described for the right medial pterygoid muscle.

Patient: Positioned in supine lying.

Therapist: Standing at the head of the patient.

Action: Support and stabilize the patient's occiput with your left hand using a football hold, cradling the posterior aspect of the occiput with your left biceps and forearm. Place the web space between your right thumb and index finger on the anterior aspect of the patient's mandible and use your right hand to open, retrude and laterally glide the mandible to the right. Both the stabilizing hand and the hand moving the body part sense the tension in the muscle and barrier. Assess the amount of range and the end feel and note the reproduction of any symptoms. Repeat this test on the contralateral side and compare the two results.

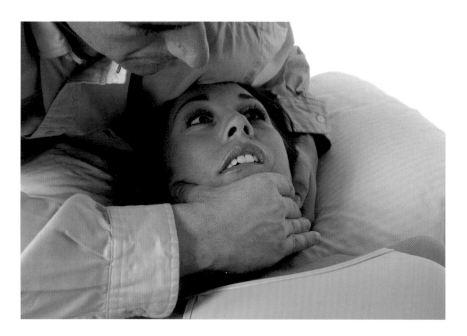

Medial Pterygoid

Technique 3

Technique described for the right medial pterygoid muscle.

Patient: Positioned in sitting.

Therapist: Standing on the left side of the patient.

Action: Support and stabilize the patient's occiput with your right hand using a football hold, cradling the posterior aspect of the occiput with your right biceps and forearm. Place the web space between your left thumb and index finger on the anterior aspect of the patient's mandible and use your left hand to open, retrude and laterally glide the mandible to the right. Both the stabilizing hand and the hand moving the body part sense the tension in the muscle and barrier. Assess the amount of range and the end feel and note the reproduction of any symptoms. Repeat this test on the contralateral side and compare the two results.

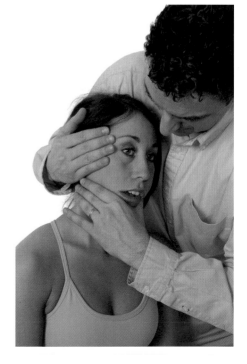

Lateral Pterygoid

Technique 1

Technique described for the right lateral pterygoid muscle.

Patient: Positioned in supine lying with the knees flexed.

Therapist: Standing on the left side of the bed.

Action: Support and stabilize the patient's occiput with your right hand using a football hold, cradling the posterior aspect of the occiput with your right biceps and forearm. Place the web space between your left thumb and index finger on the anterior aspect of the patient's mandible and use your left hand to close, retrude and laterally glide the mandible to the right. Both the stabilizing hand and the hand moving the body part sense the tension in the muscle and barrier. Assess the amount of range and the end feel and note the reproduction of any symptoms. Repeat this test on the contralateral side and compare the two results.

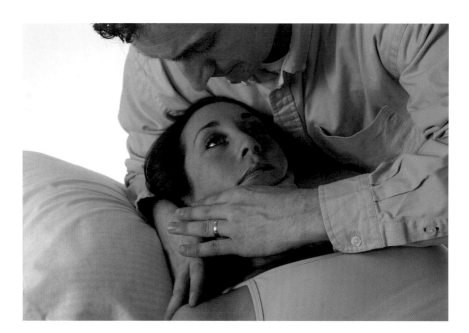

Lateral Pterygoid

Technique 2

Technique described for the right lateral pterygoid
muscle.

Patient: Positioned in sitting.

Therapist: Standing on the left side of the patient.

Action: Support and stabilize the patient's occiput with
your right hand using a football hold, cradling the
posterior aspect of the occiput with your right biceps
and forearm. Place the web space between your left
thumb and index finger on the anterior aspect of the
patient's mandible and use your left hand to close,
retrude and laterally glide the mandible to the right.
Both the stabilizing hand and the hand moving the
body part sense the tension in the muscle and barrier. Assess the amount of range and the end feel and
note the reproduction of any symptoms. Repeat this
test on the contralateral
side and compare the
two results.

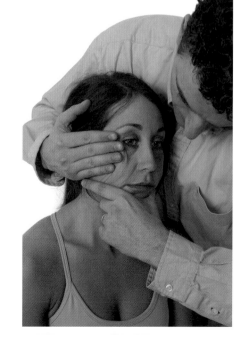

Masseter

Technique 1
Technique described for the right masseter muscle.

Patient: Positioned in supine lying with the knees flexed.

Therapist: Standing on the left side of the bed.

Action: Support and stabilize the patient's occiput with
   your right hand using a football hold, cradling the
   posterior aspect of the occiput with your right biceps
   and forearm and palpating the muscle attachment
   with your thumb. Place the web space between your
   left thumb and index finger on the anterior aspect
   of the patient's mandible and use your thumb and
   index finger to open and protrude the right side
   of the mandible. Both the stabilizing hand and the
   hand moving the body part sense the tension in the
   muscle and barrier. Assess the amount of range and
   the end feel and note the reproduction of any symptoms. Repeat this test on the contralateral side and
   compare the two results.

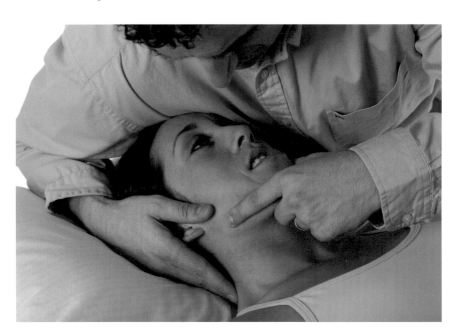

Masseter

Technique 2
Technique described for the right masseter muscle.

Patient: Positioned in supine lying with the knees flexed.

Therapist: Standing on the left side of the bed with a non-latex glove on the left hand.

Action: Support and stabilize the patient's occiput with your right hand using a football hold, cradling the posterior aspect of the occiput with your right biceps and forearm. Grasp the patient's mandible by placing your left thumb along their molars and your left index finger on the inferior aspect of the mandible. Use your left thumb and index finger to open and retrude the right side of the mandible. Assess the amount of range and the end feel and note the reproduction of any symptoms. Repeat this test on the contralateral side and compare the two results.

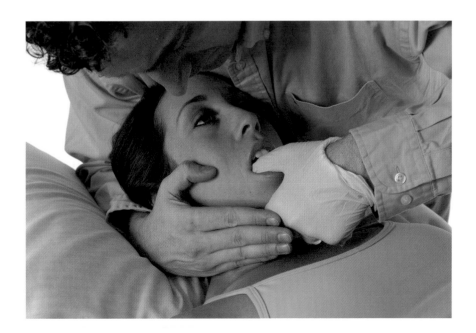

Masseter

Technique 3

Technique described for the right masseter muscle.

Patient: Positioned in sitting.

Therapist: Standing on the left side of the patient.

Action: Support and stabilize the patient's occiput with your right hand using a football hold, cradling the posterior aspect of the occiput with your right biceps and forearm and palpating the muscle attachment with your fingers. Place the web space between your left thumb and index finger on the anterior aspect of the patient's mandible and use your left hand to open and protrude the right side of the mandible. Both the stabilizing hand and the hand moving the body part sense the tension in the muscle and barrier. Assess the amount of range and the end feel and note the reproduction of any symptoms. Repeat this test on the contralateral side and compare the two results.

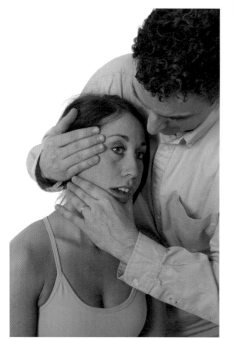

Masseter

Technique 4

Technique described for the right masseter muscle.

Patient: Positioned in sitting.

Therapist: Standing on the left side of the patient with a non-latex glove on the left hand.

Action: Support and stabilize the patient's occiput with your right hand using a football hold, cradling the posterior aspect of the occiput with your right biceps and forearm. Grasp the patient's mandible by placing your left thumb along their molars and your left index finger on the inferior aspect of the mandible. Use your left thumb and index finger to open and retrude the right side of the mandible. Both the stabilizing hand and the hand moving the body part sense the tension in the muscle and barrier. Assess the amount of range and the end feel and note the reproduction of any symptoms. Repeat this test on the contralateral side and compare the two results.

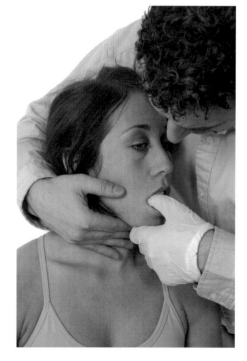

Temporalis

Technique 1
Technique described for the right temporalis muscle.

Patient: Positioned in supine lying with the knees flexed.

Therapist: Standing on the left side of the bed with a non-latex glove on the left hand.

Action: Support and stabilize the patient's occiput with your right hand using a football hold, cradling the posterior aspect of the occiput with your right biceps and forearm. Grasp the patient's mandible by placing your left thumb along their molars and your left index finger on the inferior aspect of the mandible. Use your left thumb and index finger to open, protrude and laterally deviate the mandible to the left. Both the stabilizing hand and the hand moving the body part sense the tension in the muscle and barrier. Assess the amount of range and the end feel and note the reproduction of any symptoms. Repeat this test on the contralateral side and compare the two results.

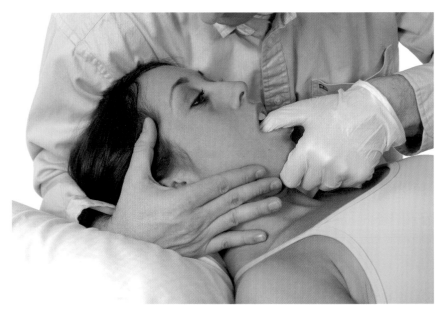

Temporalis

Technique 2

Technique described for the right temporalis muscle.

Patient: Positioned in sitting or long sitting.

Therapist: Standing on the left side of the patient with a non-latex glove on the left hand.

Action: Support and stabilize the patient's occiput with your right hand using a football hold, cradling the posterior aspect of the occiput with your right biceps and forearm. Grasp the patient's mandible by placing your left thumb on their right lower teeth and your left index finger cradled under the inferior aspect of the right angle of the mandible. Use your left thumb and index finger to open, protrude and laterally deviate the patient's right mandible to the left. Both the stabilizing hand and the hand moving the body part sense the tension in the muscle and barrier. Assess the amount of range and the end feel and note the reproduc-tion of any symptoms. Repeat this test on the contralateral side and compare the two results.

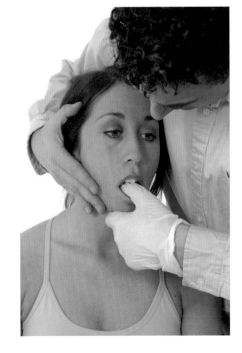

THE THORACIC SPINE

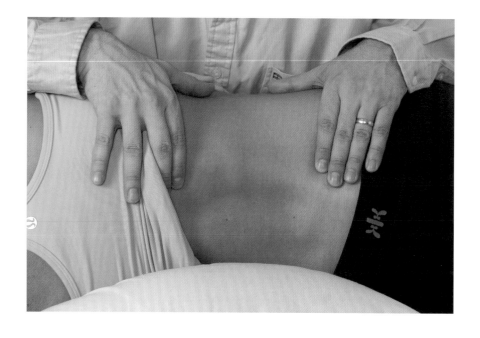

Rhomboid Major and Minor

Technique 1
Technique described for the right rhomboid major and minor muscles.

Patient: Positioned in prone lying with their hands resting under their forehead.

Therapist: Standing on the left side of the bed.

Action: The position of the patient's arms allows the scapulae to rotate upward so that the glenoid is facing superiorly. Stabilize the spinous processes of C7 to T5 with the palmar aspect of your right hand. Employing a cross-hand technique, use your left hand to depress and protract the medial border of the patient's right scapula. Both the stabilizing hand and the hand moving the body part sense the tension in the muscle and barrier. Assess the amount of range and the end feel and note the reproduction of any symptoms. Repeat this test on the contralateral side and compare the two results.

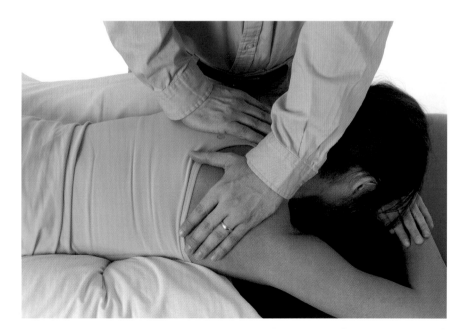

Rhomboid Major and Minor

Technique 2

Technique described for the right rhomboid major and minor muscles.

Patient: Positioned in left side lying with a pillow between the knees.

Therapist: Standing on the left side of the bed, facing the patient.

Action: Using your left hand, grasp the inferior aspect of the medial and lateral border of the right scapula. Grasp the superior aspect with your right hand. Depress, protract and upwardly rotate the right scapula so that the glenoid faces superiorly. Both the stabilizing hand and the hand moving the body part sense the tension in the muscle and barrier. Assess the amount of range and the end feel and note the reproduction of any symptoms. Repeat this test on the contralateral side and compare the two results.

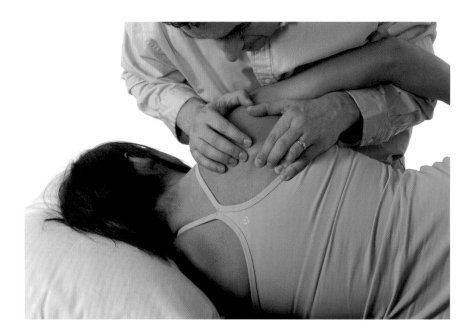

Erector Spinae

Technique 1
Technique described for the bilateral erector spinae muscles.

Patient: Positioned in side lying.

Therapist: Standing in front of the patient.

Action: Stabilize the ribs with your right hand. Use your left hand to maximally flex the thoracic and lumbar spine regions via the hips and innominates to bias the erector spinae muscles bilaterally. Both the stabilizing hand and the hand moving the body part sense the tension in the muscle and barrier. Assess the amount of range and the end feel and note the reproduction of any symptoms. Repeat this test on the contralateral side and compare the two results.

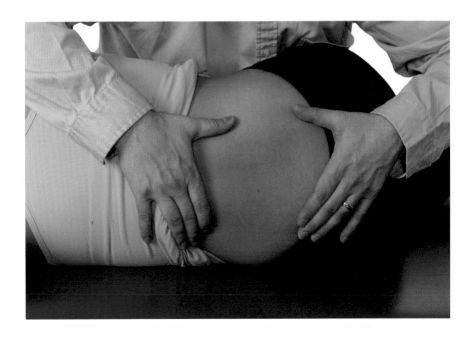

Erector Spinae

Technique 2

Technique described for the right erector spinae
muscles.

Patient: Positioned in left side lying with the right
shoulder girdle maximally flexed and horizontally
adducted overhead and a towel roll or pillow positioned under the left side of the lumbar spine.

Therapist: Standing in front of the patient.

Action: Stabilize the right ribs with your right hand.
Maximally flex the thoracic and lumbar spine regions
via the right hip and innominate with the left hand.
Add left side flexion of the trunk via the innominate
to bias the right erector spinae musculature. Both the
stabilizing hand and the hand moving the body part
sense the tension in the muscle and barrier. Assess
the amount of range and the end feel and note the
reproduction of any symptoms. Repeat this test on
the contralateral side and compare the two results.

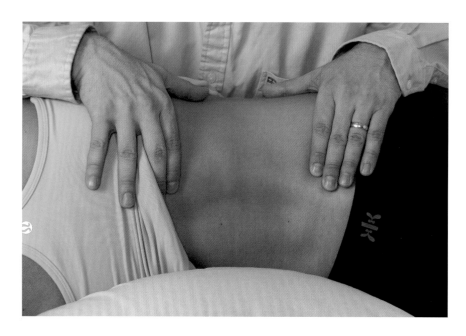

THE SHOULDER

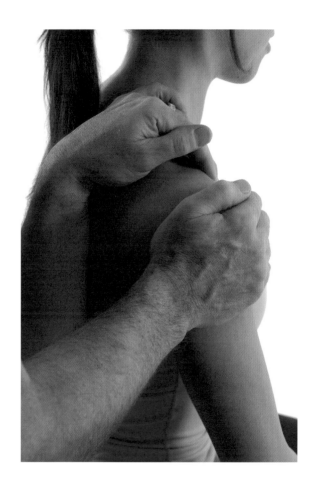

Deltoid—Anterior Fibers

Technique 1
Technique described for the right deltoid muscle.

Patient: Positioned in supine lying with the knees flexed and the right arm extending over the edge of the bed.

Therapist: Standing on the right side of the bed.

Action: Support and stabilize the superior and anterior aspect of the patient's right clavicle with your left thumb and index finger. Use your right hand to grasp the right humerus at mid-shaft, inferior to the deltoid tuberosity, and horizontally extend, externally rotate and adduct the patient's right arm. Both the stabilizing hand and the hand moving the body part sense the tension in the muscle and barrier. Assess the amount of range and the end feel and note the reproduction of any symptoms. Repeat this test on the contralateral side and compare the two results.

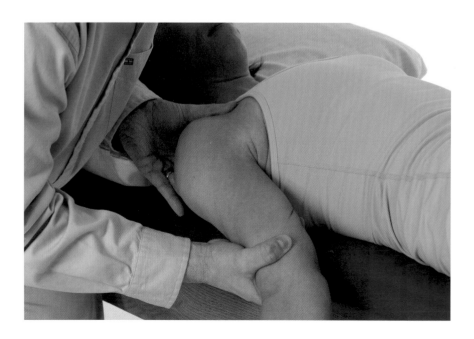

Deltoid—Anterior Fibers

Technique 2

Technique described for the right deltoid muscle.

Patient: Positioned in sitting.

Therapist: Standing on the right side of the patient.

Action: Use your left thumb and index finger to support and stabilize the superior and anterior aspect of the patient's right clavicle. With your right hand, grasp the patient's right humerus at mid-shaft, inferior to the deltoid tuberosity, and horizontally extend, externally rotate and adduct their right arm. Both the stabilizing hand and the hand moving the body part sense the tension in the muscle and barrier. Assess the amount of range and the end feel and note the reproduction of any symptoms. Repeat this test on the contralateral side and compare the two results.

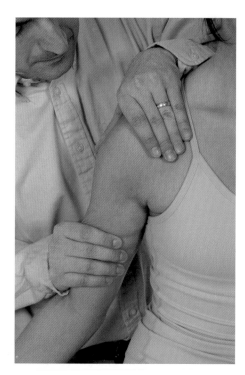

Deltoid—Middle Fibers

Technique 1
Technique described for the right deltoid muscle.

Patient: Positioned in left side lying with a pillow between the flexed knees and the right arm resting at their side.

Therapist: Standing on the left side of the bed, facing the patient.

Action: Place a rolled towel under the superior aspect of the patient's right axilla, putting the patient's right shoulder in a slightly abducted position. Use your right thumb and index finger to support and stabilize the superior aspect of the right acromion process. Then, with your left hand, grasp the patient's right humerus at mid-shaft, inferior to the deltoid tuberosity, and adduct their right arm. Both the stabilizing hand and the hand moving the body part sense the tension in the muscle and barrier. Assess the amount of range and the end feel and note the reproduction of any symptoms. Repeat this test on the contralateral side and compare the two results.

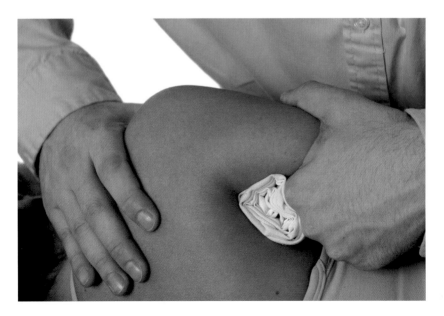

Deltoid—Middle Fibers

Technique 2
Technique described for the right deltoid muscle.

Patient: Positioned in sitting.

Therapist: Standing on the right side of the patient.

Action: Place a rolled towel under the superior aspect of the patient's right axilla, putting the patient's right shoulder in a slightly abducted position. With your left thumb and index finger, support and stabilize the superior aspect of the patient's right acromion process. Then use your right hand to grasp the patient's right humerus at mid-shaft, inferior to the deltoid tuberosity, and adduct their right arm. Both the stabilizing hand and the hand moving the body part sense the tension in the muscle and barrier. Assess the amount of range and the end feel and note the reproduction of any symptoms. Repeat this test on the contralateral side and compare the two results.

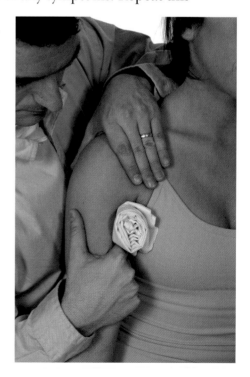

Deltoid—Posterior Fibers

Technique 1
Technique described for the right deltoid muscle.

Patient: Positioned in left side lying with the right arm resting over the edge of the bed.

Therapist: Standing on the left side of the bed.

Action: Using your right thumb and index finger, support and stabilize the patient's right acromion process and spine of the scapula. With your left hand, grasp the right humerus at mid-shaft, inferior to the deltoid tuberosity, and horizontally flex, internally rotate and adduct the patient's right arm. Both the stabilizing hand and the hand moving the body part sense the tension in the muscle and barrier. Assess the amount of range and the end feel and note the reproduction of any symptoms. Repeat this test on the contralateral side and compare the two results.

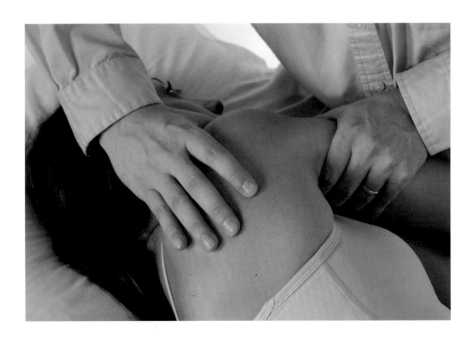

Deltoid—Posterior Fibers

Technique 2
Technique described for the right deltoid muscle.

Patient: Positioned in sitting.

Therapist: Standing on the right side of the patient.

Action: Using your right thumb and index finger, support and stabilize the patient's right acromion process and spine of the scapula. With your left hand, grasp the right humerus at mid-shaft, inferior to the deltoid tuberosity, and horizontally flex, internally rotate and adduct the patient's right arm. Both the stabilizing hand and the hand moving the body part sense the tension in the muscle and barrier. Assess the amount of range and the end feel and note the reproduction of any symptoms. Repeat this test on the contralateral side and compare the two results.

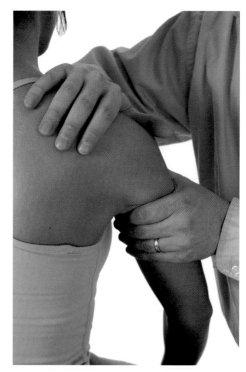

Supraspinatus

Technique 1
Technique described for the right supraspinatus muscle.

Patient: Positioned in left side lying with a pillow between the flexed knees and with their right arm resting at their side.

Therapist: Standing on the left side of the bed, facing the patient.

Action: Place a rolled towel under the superior aspect of the patient's right axilla, putting the patient's right shoulder in a slightly abducted position. Using your right thumb and index finger, support and stabilize the superior and medial aspect of the patient's right scapula. With your left hand, grasp the patient's right humerus at mid-shaft, inferior to the deltoid tuberosity, and adduct the right arm. Slight internal rotation of the right humerus may also be added to further

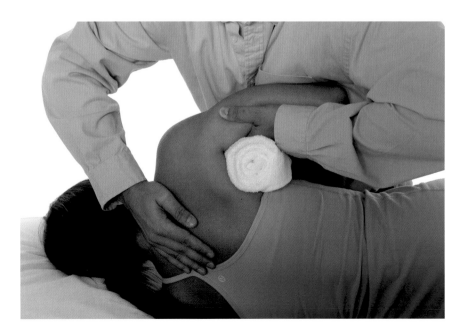

tension the right supraspinatus muscle. Both the stabilizing hand and the hand moving the body part sense the tension in the muscle and barrier. Assess the amount of range and the end feel and note the reproduction of any symptoms. Repeat this test on the contralateral side and compare the two results.

Supraspinatus

Technique 2

Technique described for the right supraspinatus
muscle.

Patient: Positioned in sitting.

Therapist: Standing on the right side of the patient.

Action: Place a rolled towel under the superior aspect
of the patient's right axilla, putting the patient's right
shoulder in a slightly abducted position. Using your
right thumb and index finger, support and stabilize
the superior and medial aspect of the patient's right
scapula. With your left hand, grasp the patient's right
humerus at mid-shaft, inferior to the deltoid tuberosity, and adduct and internally rotate the patient's
right arm. Both the stabilizing hand and the hand
moving the body part sense the tension in the muscle
and barrier. Assess the amount of range and the end
feel and note the reproduction of any symptoms.
Repeat this test on the contralateral side and compare the two results.

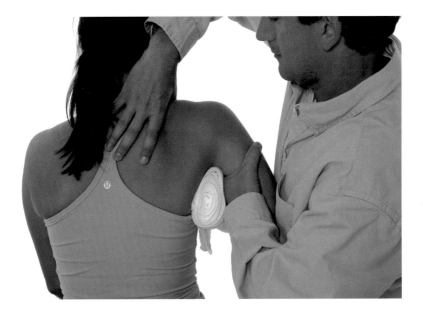

Infraspinatus

Technique 1
Technique described for the right infraspinatus muscle.

Patient: Positioned in supine lying with the knees flexed.

Therapist: Standing on the right side of the bed.

Action: Abduct the patient's right shoulder to 90° and rest their right elbow and upper arm on the bed. Stabilize the patient's right scapula with your right hand, placing your right thumb in the axillary fold to stabilize the infraglenoid tubercle while your fingers stabilize the anterior aspect of the shoulder. With your left hand, grasp the right distal forearm and internally rotate the patient's right arm. Both the stabilizing hand and the hand moving the body part sense the tension in the muscle and barrier. Assess the amount of range and the end feel and note the reproduction of any symptoms. Repeat this test on the contralateral side and compare the two results.

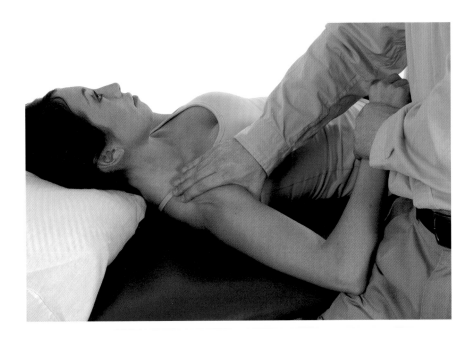

Infraspinatus

Technique 2

Technique described for the right infraspinatus muscle.

Patient: Positioned in supine lying with the knees flexed.

Therapist: Standing at the head of the bed.

Action: Abduct the patient's right shoulder to 90° and rest their right elbow and upper arm on the bed. Stabilize the patient's right shoulder with your left hand tucked under the scapula and your left thumb over the coracoid process. Use your right hand to grasp the right distal forearm and internally rotate the patient's right arm. Both the stabilizing hand and the hand moving the body part sense the tension in the muscle and barrier. Assess the amount of range and the end feel and note the reproduction of any symptoms. Repeat this test on the contralateral side and compare the two results.

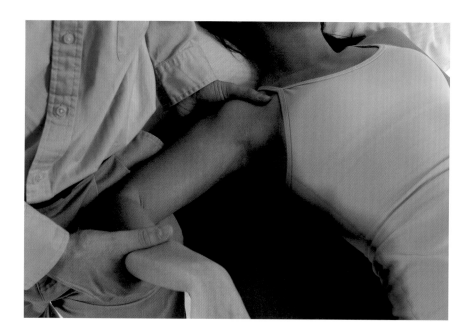

Subscapularis

Technique described for the right subscapularis muscle.

Patient: Positioned in supine lying with the knees flexed.

Therapist: Standing on the right side of the bed.

Action: Abduct the patient's right shoulder to 90° and rest their right elbow and upper arm on the bed. Stabilize the patient's right scapula with your right hand, with your thumb in the axillary fold to stabilize the infraglenoid tubercle and with your fingers cupped over the anterior and superior aspect. With your left hand, grasp the right distal forearm and externally rotate the patient's right arm. Both the stabilizing hand and the hand moving the body part sense the tension in the muscle and barrier. Assess the amount of range and the end feel and note the reproduction of any symptoms. Repeat this test on the contralateral side and compare the two results.

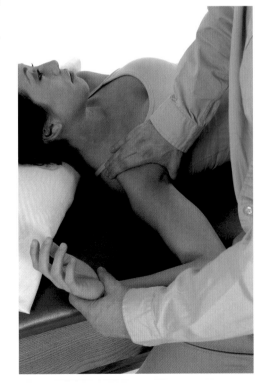

Teres Minor

Technique described for the right teres minor muscle.

Patient: Positioned in supine lying with the knees flexed.

Therapist: Standing on the right side of the bed.

Action: Flex the patient's right shoulder to 180°.
Stabilize the lateral border of the patient's right
scapula with your right hand. With your left hand,
grasp the patient's right distal forearm and internally
rotate the arm. Both the stabilizing hand and the
hand moving the body part sense the tension in
the muscle and barrier. Assess the amount of range
and the end feel and note the reproduction of any
symptoms. Repeat this test on the contralateral side
and compare the two results.

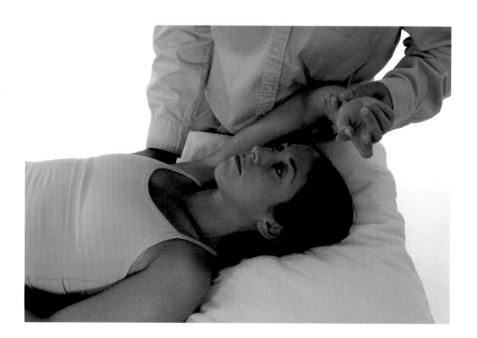

Teres Major

Technique described for the right teres major muscle.

Patient: Positioned in supine lying with the knees flexed.

Therapist: Standing on the right side of the bed.

Action: Flex the patient's right shoulder to 180°. Stabilize the lateral border of the patient's right scapula
with your right hand. With your left hand, grasp
the patient's right proximal forearm and externally
rotate the arm. Both the stabilizing hand and the
hand moving the body part sense the tension in the
muscle and barrier. Assess the amount of range and
the end feel and note the reproduction of any symptoms. Repeat this test on the contralateral side and
compare the two results.

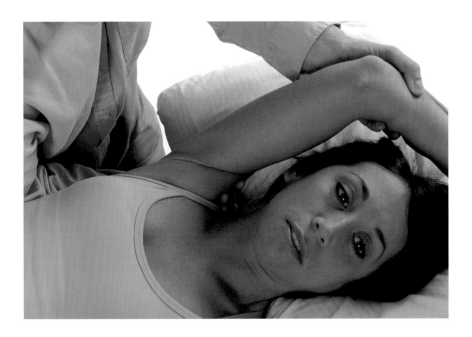

Pectoralis Major and Minor

General Test

Technique described for the right pectoralis major and pectoralis minor muscles.

Patient: Positioned in sitting.

Therapist: Standing behind and on the right side of the patient.

Action: Stabilize the patient's right scapula with your left hand or forearm. With your right hand, grasp the patient's right humerus and glide the head of the humerus posteriorly. Both the stabilizing hand and the hand moving the body part sense the tension in the pectoralis major muscle and barrier. Assess the amount of range and the end feel and note the reproduction of any symptoms. Repeat this test on the contralateral side and compare the two results.

The left hand can then be moved to stabilize the upper to mid thoracic spine. With your right hand,

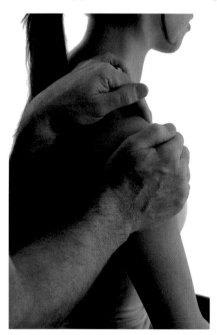

grasp the patient's coracoid process and glide the scapula posteriorly. Both the stabilizing hand and the hand moving the body part sense the tension in the pectoralis minor muscle and barrier. Assess the amount of range and the end feel and note the reproduction of any symptoms. Repeat this test on the contralateral side and compare the two results.

Pectoralis Major

Technique 1 – Clavicular Fibers

Technique described for the right pectoralis major muscle.

Patient: Positioned in supine lying with the knees flexed.

Therapist: Standing at the head of the bed.

Action: Abduct the patient's right shoulder to 45° and rest their right elbow and upper arm over the edge of the bed. Stabilize the inferior aspect of the patient's right clavicle with the palm of your left hand. Use your right hand to grasp the right distal aspect of the patient's right humerus and horizontally extend, externally rotate and abduct the right arm. Both the stabilizing hand and the hand moving the body part sense the tension in the muscle and barrier. Assess the amount of range and the end feel and note the reproduction of any symptoms. Repeat this test on the contralateral side and compare the two results.

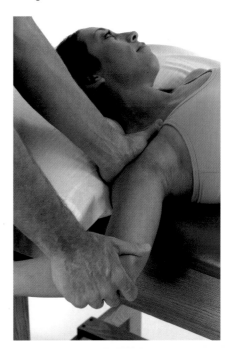

Pectoralis Major

Technique 2 – Sternal Fibers
Technique described for the right pectoralis major
muscle.

Patient: Positioned in supine lying with the knees flexed.

Therapist: Standing at the head of the bed.

Action: Abduct the patient's right shoulder to 90° and
    rest their right elbow and upper arm over the edge
    of the bed. Stabilize the right lateral border of the
    patient's sternum with the palm of your left hand.
    Use your right hand to grasp the right distal aspect of
    the patient's right humerus and horizontally extend,
    externally rotate and abduct the right arm. Both the
    stabilizing hand and the hand moving the body part
    sense the tension in the muscle and barrier. Assess
    the amount of range and the end feel and note the
    reproduction of any symptoms. Repeat this test on
    the contralateral side and compare the two results.

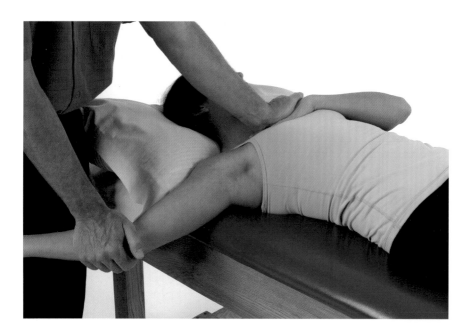

Pectoralis Major

Technique 3 - Sternocostal Fibers
Technique described for the right pectoralis major muscle.

Patient: Positioned in supine lying with the knees flexed.

Therapist: Standing at the head of the bed.

Action: Abduct the patient's right shoulder to 120° and rest their right elbow and upper arm over the edge of the bed. Stabilize the right lateral border of the patient's sternum and chondral area of the 6th to 8th ribs with the palm of your left hand. Use your right hand to grasp the right distal aspect of the patient's right humerus to horizontally extend, externally rotate and abduct the right arm. Both the stabilizing hand and the hand moving the body part sense the tension in the muscle and barrier. Assess the amount of range and the end feel and note the reproduction of any symptoms. Repeat this test on the contralateral side and compare the two results.

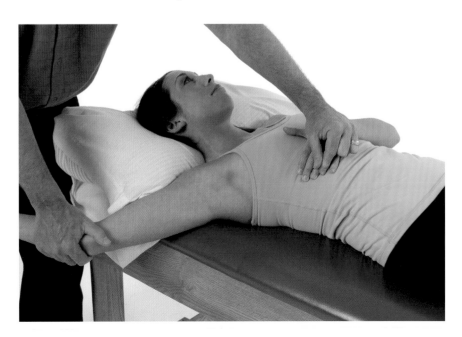

Pectoralis Minor

Technique 1

Technique described for the right pectoralis minor muscle.

Patient: Positioned in supine lying with the knees flexed.

Therapist: Standing on the right side of the bed.

Action: Note the distance between the lateral border of the spine of the right scapula and the top of the bed. If there is tightness in the pectoralis minor, this distance may be greater than 1 inch (2.54 cm). Repeat this test on the contralateral side and compare the two results.

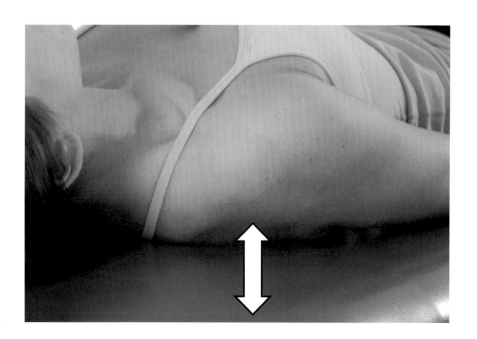

Pectoralis Minor

Technique 2

Technique described for the right pectoralis minor
muscle.

Patient: Positioned in supine lying with the knees flexed.

Therapist: Standing on the right side of the bed.

Action: Stabilize the anterior aspect of the patient's
3rd, 4th and 5th ribs with your right hand. Use the
palmar aspect of your left hand to cup the right coracoid process and anterior aspect of the scapula. Glide
the patient's right scapula superiorly and posteriorly.
Both the stabilizing hand and the hand moving the
body part sense the tension in the muscle and barrier. Assess the amount of range and the end feel and
note the reproduction of any symptoms. Repeat this
test on the contralateral side and compare the two
results.

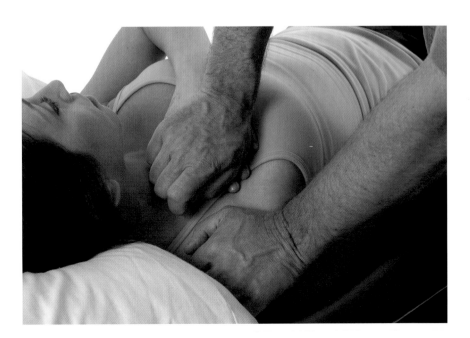

Subclavius

Technique described for the right subclavius muscle.

Patient: Positioned in supine lying with the knees flexed.

Therapist: Standing on the right side of the bed.

Action: Stabilize the right 1st rib using the palmar aspect of your right hand. Use your left thumb to elevate and posteriorly translate the right clavicle. Both the stabilizing hand and the hand moving the body part sense the tension in the muscle and barrier. Assess the amount of range and the end feel and note the reproduction of any symptoms. Repeat this test on the contralateral side and compare the two results.

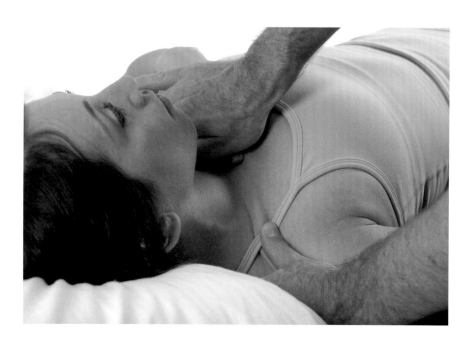

THE ELBOW

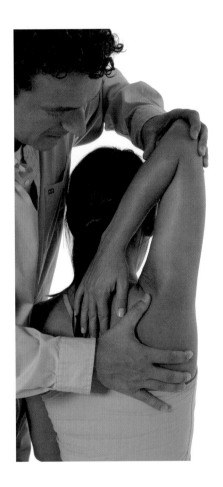

Biceps Brachii

Technique 1

Technique described for the right biceps brachii muscle.

Patient: Positioned in supine lying with the knees flexed.

Therapist: Standing on the right side of the bed.

Action: Rest the patient's right shoulder and elbow over the edge of the bed. Stabilize their right shoulder with your right hand, placing your right thumb in the axillary fold to stabilize the infraglenoid tubercle of the right scapula and with your fingers cupped over the anterior aspect of the right shoulder and coracoid process. Use your left hand to grasp the proximal aspect of the patient's right forearm to extend the humerus and extend and pronate the elbow and forearm. Both the stabilizing hand and the hand moving the body part sense the tension in the muscle and barrier. Assess the amount of range and the end feel and note the reproduction of any symptoms. Repeat this test on the contralateral side and compare the two results.

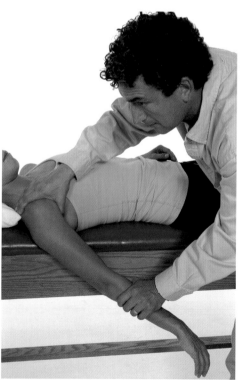

Biceps Brachii

Technique 2

Technique described for the right biceps brachii
muscle.

Patient: Positioned in sitting.

Therapist: Standing behind the right side of the patient.

Action: Stabilize the anterior and superior aspect of
the patient's right shoulder and the posterior aspect
of their right scapula with your left hand cupped
over the anterior and posterior aspect of the right
shoulder and coracoid process. Your left forearm
rests against the posterior aspect of the patient's
right scapula. With your right hand, grasp the
proximal aspect of the patient's right forearm to
extend the right shoulder and extend and pronate
the right elbow and
forearm. Both the
stabilizing hand
and the hand mov-
ing the body part
sense the tension
in the muscle and
barrier. Assess the
amount of range
and the end feel
and note the
reproduction of any
symptoms. Repeat
this test on the
contralateral side
and compare the
two results.

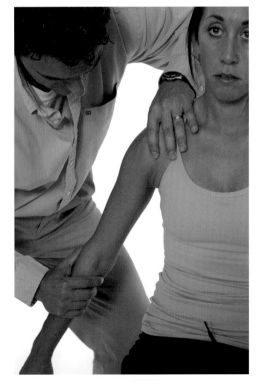

Coracobrachialis

Technique described for the right coracobrachialis
muscle.

Patient: Positioned in supine lying with the knees flexed.

Therapist: Standing on the right side of the bed.

Action: Rest the patient's right shoulder and elbow over
the edge of the bed. Stabilize their right scapula with
your right hand, placing your right thumb over the
coracoid process and your fingers cupped over the
posterior aspect of the right scapula. Uses your left
hand to grasp the right distal aspect of the patient's
upper arm and horizontally extend and abduct the
humerus. Both the stabilizing hand and the hand
moving the body part sense the tension in the muscle
and barrier. Assess the amount of range and the end
feel and note the reproduction of any symptoms.
Repeat this test on the contralateral side and
compare the two results.

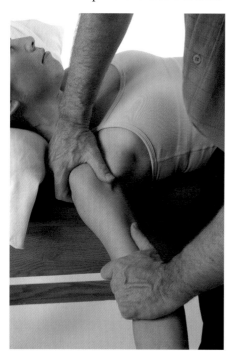

Brachialis

Technique described for the right brachialis muscle.

Patient: Positioned in supine lying with the knees flexed.

Therapist: Standing on the right side of the bed.

Action: Use your left hand to grasp the patient's right humerus at mid-shaft and stabilize the anterior aspect of the right arm. You may also use your left forearm to stabilize the anterior aspect of the patient's right shoulder. With your right hand, grasp the distal aspect of the patient's right forearm and extend the right elbow and forearm. Both the stabilizing hand and the hand moving the body part sense the tension in the muscle and barrier. Assess the amount of range and the end feel and note the reproduction of any symptoms. Repeat this test on the contralateral side and compare the two results.

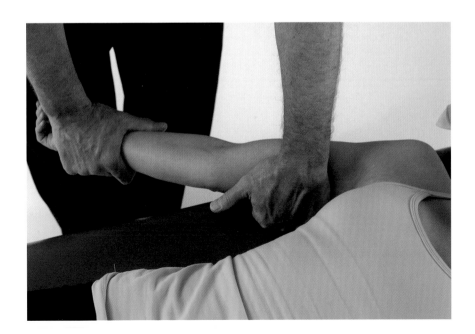

Triceps Brachii

Technique described for the right triceps brachii muscle.

Patient: Positioned in sitting.

Therapist: Standing behind the patient.

Action: Use your right hand to stabilize the lateral border of the patient's right scapula. With your left hand, grasp the proximal aspect of the patient's right forearm to flex the right shoulder and flex the right elbow overhead. Both the stabilizing hand and the hand moving the body part sense the tension in the muscle and barrier. Assess the amount of range and the end feel and note the reproduction of any symptoms. Repeat this test on the contralateral side and compare the two results.

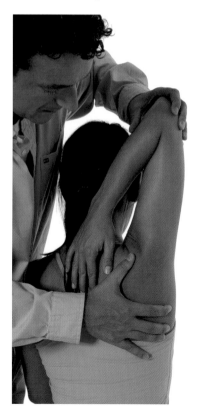

Supinator

Technique described for the right supinator muscle.

Patient: Positioned in left side lying with a pillow between flexed knees and their right arm resting at their side.

Therapist: Standing on the right side of the bed.

Action: With your right hand, extend the patient's right elbow and pronate their right forearm. With your right thumb, apply an anterior glide to the proximal aspect of the right radius. Both the stabilizing hand and the hand moving the body part sense the tension in the muscle and barrier. Assess the amount of range and the end feel and note the reproduction of any symptoms. Repeat this test on the contralateral side and compare the two results.

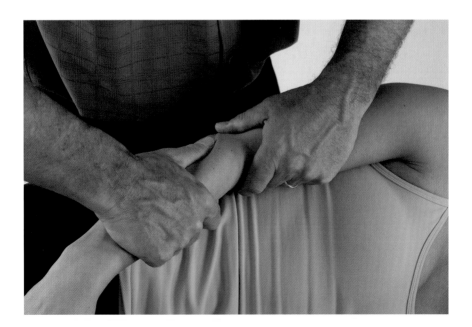

Pronator Teres

Technique described for the right pronator teres muscle.

Patient: Positioned in supine lying with the knees flexed.

Therapist: Standing on the right side of the bed.

Action: Use your left hand to stabilize the patient's distal right humerus, monitoring tension in the pronator teres muscle with your left fingers. Use your right hand to extend the patient's right elbow and supinate the right forearm. Both the stabilizing hand and the hand moving the body part sense the tension in the muscle and barrier. Assess the amount of range and the end feel and note the reproduction of any symptoms. Repeat this test on the contralateral side and compare the two results.

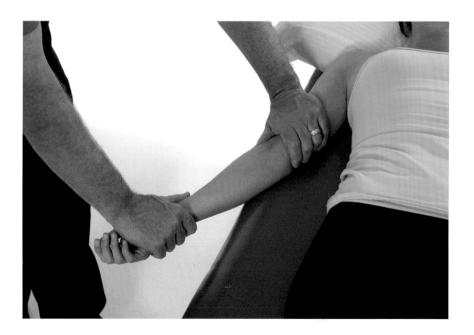

Brachioradialis

Technique described for the right brachioradialis muscle.

Patient: Positioned in supine lying with the knees flexed.

Therapist: Standing on the right side of the bed.

Action: Use your left hand to grasp and stabilize the patient's distal right humerus. Keep the patient's shoulder in a flexed position, and use your right hand to extend their right elbow and pronate the forearm. Both the stabilizing hand and the hand moving the body part sense the tension in the muscle and barrier. Assess the amount of range and the end feel and note the reproduction of any symptoms. Repeat this test on the contralateral side and compare the two results.

This same technique can also be used in supinating the patient's forearm instead of pronating it. As usual, the same test is repeated on the contralateral side and compared.

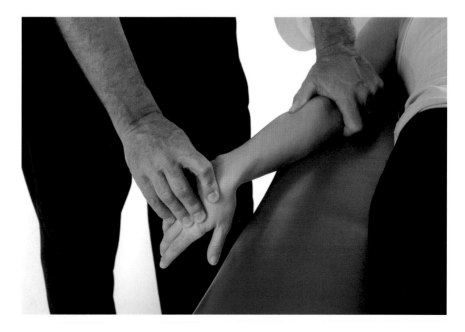

THE WRIST AND HAND

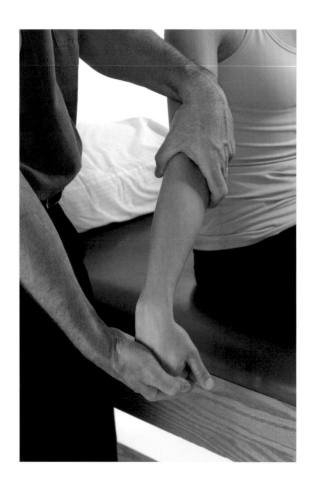

Extensor Carpi Radialis Longus

Technique described for the right extensor carpi radialis longus muscle.

Patient: Positioned in supine lying with the knees flexed.

Therapist: Standing on the right side of the bed.

Action: Use your left hand to grasp and stabilize the patient's distal right humerus. With your right hand, grasp the dorsal surface of the right wrist and extend the patient's right elbow, flex and ulnar deviate the right wrist and flex the 2nd metacarpal. Both the stabilizing hand and the hand moving the body part sense the tension in the muscle and barrier. Assess the amount of range and the end feel and note the reproduction of any symptoms. Repeat this test on the contralateral side and compare the two results.

Note also the reproduction of any dural symptoms. To differentiate between neuromeningeal tissue and the patient's muscle, add various sensitizing movements of the upper extremities and note any change in the amount of range, the end feel and the symptoms produced.

This same technique can also be used with the patient positioned in sitting.

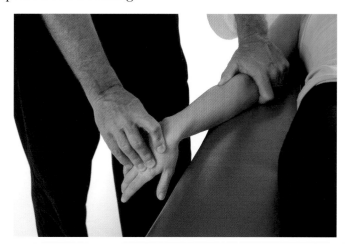

Extensor Carpi Radialis Brevis

Technique described for the right extensor carpi radialis brevis muscle.

Patient: Positioned in supine lying with the knees flexed.

Therapist: Standing on the right side of the bed.

Action: Use your left hand to grasp and stabilize the patient's distal right humerus. With your right hand, extend the patient's right elbow, flex and ulnar deviate the right wrist and flex the 3rd metacarpal. Both the stabilizing hand and the hand moving the body part sense the tension in the muscle and barrier. Assess the amount of range and the end feel and note the reproduction of any symptoms. Repeat this test on the contralateral side and compare the two results.

Note also the reproduction of any dural symptoms. To differentiate between neuromeningeal tissue and the patient's muscle, add various sensitizing movements of the upper extremities and note any change in the amount of range, the end feel and the symptoms produced.

This same technique can also be used with the patient positioned in sitting.

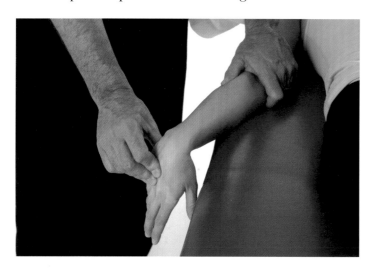

Extensor Carpi Ulnaris

Technique described for the right extensor carpi ulnaris muscle.

Patient: Positioned in sitting.

Therapist: Standing on the right hand side of the patient.

Action: Grasp and stabilize the patient's distal right humerus with your left hand. With your right hand, extend the patient's right elbow, flex and radially deviate the right wrist and flex the 5th metacarpal. Both the stabilizing hand and the hand moving the body part sense the tension in the muscle and barrier. Assess the amount of range and the end feel and note the reproduction of any symptoms. Repeat this test on the contralateral side and compare the two results.

Note also the reproduction of any dural symptoms. To differentiate between neuromeningeal tissue and the patient's muscle, add various sensitizing movements of the upper extremities and note any change in the amount of range, the end feel and the symptoms produced.

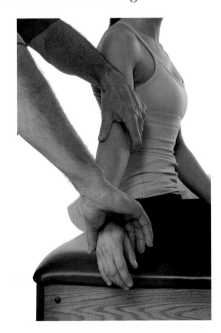

This same technique can also be used with the patient positioned in supine.

Extensor Digitorum

Technique described for the right extensor digitorum muscle.

Patient: Positioned in supine lying with the knees flexed.

Therapist: Standing on the right side of the bed.

Action: Grasp and stabilize the patient's distal right humerus with your left hand. Ask the patient to flex and make a fist with their 2nd to 5th carpometacarpal joints, their metacarpophalangeal joints and their proximal and distal interphalangeal joints. Use your right hand to hold the patient's 2nd to 5th digits in this position, then extend their right elbow and flex their right wrist. Both the stabilizing hand and the hand moving the body part sense the tension in the muscle and barrier. Assess the amount of range and the end feel and note the reproduction of any symptoms. Repeat this test on the contralateral side and compare the two results.

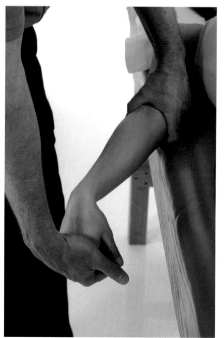

Note also the reproduction of any dural symptoms. To differentiate between neuromeningeal tissue and the patient's muscle, add various sensitizing movements of the upper extremities and note any change in the amount of range, the end feel and the symptoms produced.

This same technique can also be used with the patient positioned in sitting.

Extensor Digiti Minimi

Technique described for the right extensor digiti minimi muscle.

Patient: Positioned in supine lying with the knees flexed.

Therapist: Standing on the right side of the bed.

Action: Grasp and stabilize the patient's distal right humerus with your left hand. Ask the patient to flex their 5th carpometacarpal joint, their metacarpophalangeal joints and their proximal and distal interphalangeal joints. Use your right hand to hold the patient's 5th digit in this position, then extend their right elbow and flex their right wrist. Both the stabilizing hand and the hand moving the body part sense the tension in the muscle and barrier. Assess the amount of range and the end feel and note the reproduction of any symptoms. Repeat this test on the contralateral side and compare the two results.

Note also the reproduction of any dural symptoms. To differentiate between neuromeningeal tissue and the patient's muscle, add various sensitizing movements of the upper extremities and note any change in the amount of range, the end feel and the symptoms produced.

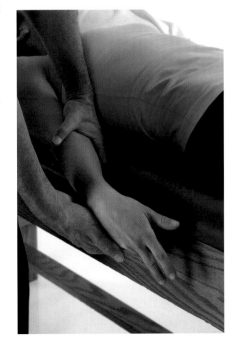

This same technique can also be used with the patient positioned in sitting.

Extensor Indicis

Technique described for the right extensor indicis muscle.

Patient: Positioned in supine lying with the knees flexed.

Therapist: Standing on the right side of the bed.

Action: Grasp and stabilize the middle of the patient's right ulna with your left hand. Ask the patient to flex their 2nd carpometacarpal joint and metacarpophalangeal joint. Use your right hand to hold the 2nd digit in this position, then flex and radially deviate the patient's right wrist. Both the stabilizing hand and the hand moving the body part sense the tension in the muscle and barrier. Assess the amount of range and the end feel and note the reproduction of any symptoms. Repeat this test on the contralateral side and compare the two results.

Note also the reproduction of any dural symptoms. To differentiate between neuromeningeal tissue

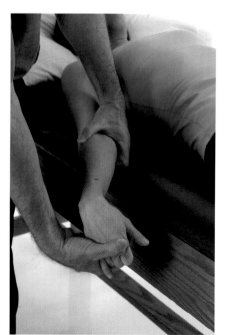

and the patient's muscle, add various sensitizing movements of the upper extremities and note any change in the amount of range, the end feel and the symptoms produced.

This same technique can also be used with the patient positioned in sitting.

Flexor Carpi Radialis

Technique described for the right flexor carpi radialis muscle.

Patient: Positioned in supine lying with the knees flexed.

Therapist: Standing on the right side of the bed.

Action: Use your left hand to stabilize the patient's distal right humerus. With your right hand, extend the patient's right elbow, extend and ulnar deviate their right wrist and extend their 2nd and 3rd metacarpals. Both the stabilizing hand and the hand moving the body part sense the tension in the muscle and barrier. Assess the amount of range and the end feel and note the reproduction of any symptoms. Repeat this test on the contralateral side and compare the two results.

Note also the reproduction of any dural symptoms. To differentiate between neuromeningeal tissue and the patient's muscle, add various sensitizing movements of the upper extremities and note any change in the amount of range, the end feel and the symptoms produced.

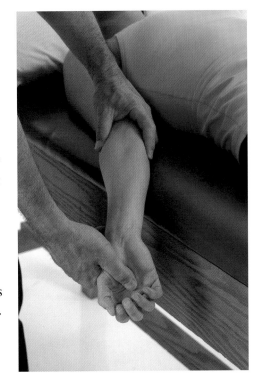

This same technique can also be used with the patient positioned in sitting using your left hand and forearm to stabilize the patient's distal right humerus.

Flexor Carpi Ulnaris

Technique described for the right flexor carpi ulnaris muscle.

Patient: Positioned in supine lying with the knees flexed.

Therapist: Standing on the right side of the bed.

Action: Use your left hand to stabilize the patient's distal right humerus. With your right hand, extend the patient's right elbow and extend and radially deviate their right wrist. Both the stabilizing hand and the hand moving the body part sense the tension in the muscle and barrier. Assess the amount of range and the end feel and note the reproduction of any symptoms. Repeat this test on the contralateral side and compare the two results.

Note also the reproduction of any dural symptoms. To differentiate between neuromeningeal tissue and the patient's muscle, add various sensitizing

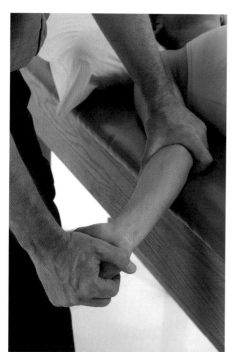

movements of the upper extremities and note any change in the amount of range, the end feel and the symptoms produced.

This same technique can also be used with the patient positioned in sitting using your left hand and forearm to stabilize the patient's distal right humerus.

Palmaris Longus

Technique described for the right palmaris longus muscle.

Patient: Positioned in supine lying with the knees flexed.

Therapist: Standing on the right side of the bed.

Action: Use your left hand and forearm to stabilize the patient's distal right humerus. With your right hand, extend the patient's right elbow and right wrist, keeping all of the fingers and the thumb of their right hand in an extended position. Both the stabilizing hand and the hand moving the body part sense the tension in the muscle and barrier. Assess the amount of range and the end feel and note the reproduction of any symptoms. Repeat this test on the contralateral side and compare the two results.

Note also the reproduction of any dural symptoms. To differentiate between neuromeningeal tissue and the patient's muscle, add various sensitizing movements of the upper extremities and note any change in the amount of range, the end feel and the symptoms produced.

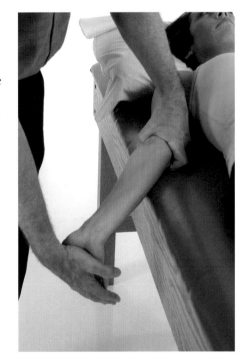

This same technique can also be used with the patient positioned in sitting using your left hand and forearm to stabilize the patient's distal right humerus.

Flexor Digitorum Superficialis

Technique described for the right flexor digitorum superficialis muscle.

Patient: Positioned in supine lying with the knees flexed.

Therapist: Standing on the right side of the bed.

Action: Use your left hand to stabilize the patient's distal right humerus. With your right hand, extend the patient's right elbow, right wrist and the proximal interphalangeal joints of the 2nd, 3rd, 4th and 5th digits, keeping the distal phalanges in a flexed position. Both the stabilizing hand and the hand moving the body part sense the tension in the muscle and barrier. Assess the amount of range and the end feel and note the reproduction of any symptoms. Repeat this test on the contralateral side and compare the two results.

Note also the reproduction of any dural symptoms. To differentiate between neuromeningeal tissue

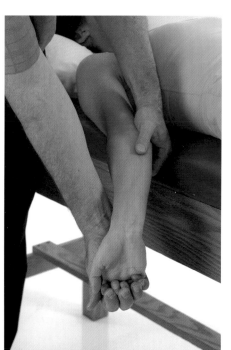

and the patient's muscle, add various sensitizing movements of the upper extremities and note any change in the amount of range, the end feel and the symptoms produced.

This same technique can also be used with the patient positioned in sitting using your left hand and forearm to stabilize the patient's distal right humerus.

Flexor Digitorum Profundus

Technique described for the right flexor digitorum profundus muscle.

Patient: Positioned in supine lying with the knees flexed.

Therapist: Standing on the right side of the bed.

Action: Use your left hand to stabilize the patient's distal right humerus and proximal right ulna. With your right hand, extend the patient's right elbow, right wrist and the proximal and distal interphalangeal joints of the 2nd, 3rd, 4th and 5th digits. Both the stabilizing hand and the hand moving the body part sense the tension in the muscle and barrier. Assess the amount of range and the end feel and note the reproduction of any symptoms. Repeat this test on the contralateral side and compare the two results.

Note also the reproduction of any dural symptoms. To differentiate between neuromeningeal tissue and the patient's muscle, add various sensitizing movements of the upper extremities and note any change in the amount of range, the end feel and the symptoms produced.

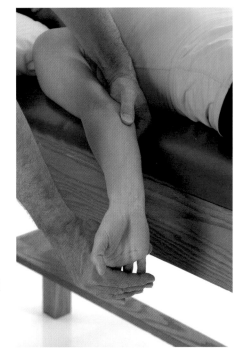

This same technique can also be used with the patient positioned in sitting using your left hand and forearm to stabilize the patient's distal right humerus and proximal right ulna.

Extensor Pollicis Longus

Technique described for the right extensor pollicis longus muscle.

Patient: Positioned in supine lying with the knees flexed.

Therapist: Standing on the right side of the bed.

Action: Use your left hand to grasp and stabilize the middle of the patient's right ulna, keeping their right wrist in a neutral position. With your right thumb, flex the 1st carpometacarpal joint, the metacarpophalangeal joint and the interphalangeal joint and adduct the 1st metacarpal. Both the stabilizing hand and the hand moving the body part sense the tension in the muscle and barrier. Assess the amount of range and the end feel and note the reproduction of any symptoms. Repeat this test on the contralateral side and compare the two results.

Note also the reproduction of any dural symptoms. To differentiate between neuromeningeal tissue

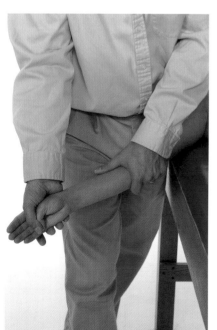

and the patient's muscle, add various sensitizing movements of the upper extremities and note any change in the amount of range, the end feel and the symptoms produced.

This same technique can also be used with the patient positioned in sitting.

Extensor Pollicis Brevis

Technique described for the right extensor pollicis brevis muscle.

Patient: Positioned in supine lying with the knees flexed.

Therapist: Standing on the right side of the bed.

Action: Use your left hand to grasp and stabilize the middle of the patient's right ulna, keeping the patient's right wrist in a neutral position. With the fingers of your right hand, flex the 1st carpometacarpal joint and metacarpophalangeal joint, keeping the 1st interphalangeal joint in a neutral position, and adduct the 1st metacarpal. Both the stabilizing hand and the hand moving the body part sense the tension in the muscle and barrier. Assess the amount of range and the end feel and note the reproduction of any symptoms. Repeat this test on the contralateral side and compare the two results.

This same technique can also be used with the patient positioned in sitting.

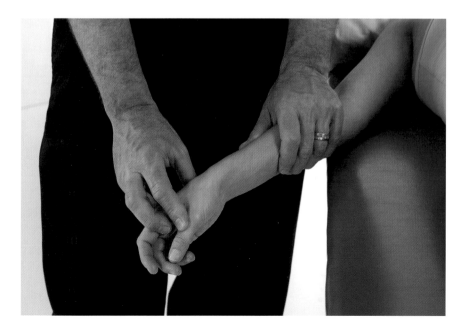

Abductor Pollicis Longus

Technique described for the right abductor pollicis longus muscle.

Patient: Positioned in supine lying with the knees flexed.

Therapist: Standing on the right side of the bed.

Action: Use your left hand to grasp and stabilize the middle of the patient's right ulna and radius, keeping their right wrist in an ulnar deviated position. With the fingers of your right hand, flex and adduct the 1st carpometacarpal joint, keeping the right 1st metacarpophalangeal joint and interphalangeal joint in a neutral position. Both the stabilizing hand and the hand moving the body part sense the tension in the muscle and barrier. Assess the amount of range and the end feel and note the reproduction of any symptoms. Repeat this test on the contralateral side and compare the two results.

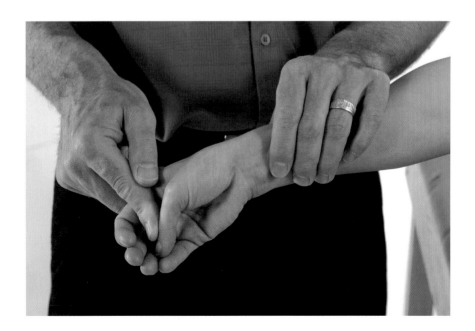

Note also the reproduction of any dural symptoms.
To differentiate between neuromeningeal tissue
and the patient's muscle, add various sensitizing
movements of the upper extremities and note any
change in the amount of range, the end feel and the
symptoms produced.

This same technique can also be used with the
patient positioned in sitting.

Flexor Pollicis Longus

Technique described for the right flexor pollicis longus muscle.

Patient: Positioned in supine lying with the knees flexed.

Therapist: Standing on the right side of the bed.

Action: Use your left hand to stabilize the patient's distal right ulna and radius. Ulnar deviate the patient's right wrist with the fingers and thumb of your left hand. With the index finger of your right hand extend the 1st carpometacarpal joint, the metacarpophalangeal joint and the interphalangeal joints. Assess the amount of range and the end feel and note the reproduction of any symptoms. Repeat this test on the contralateral side and compare the two results.

This same technique can also be used with the patient positioned in sitting.

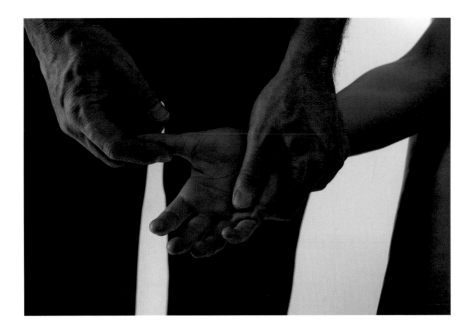

References

Butler, D. 1991. *Mobilization of the Nervous System*. New York: Churchill Livingstone.

Butler, D. (2000). *The Sensitive Nervous System*. Adelaide, Australia: Noigroup Publications.

Evjenth, O. 1988. *Muscle Stretching in Manual Therapy: A Clinical Manual – The Extremities*, vol. 1. Alfta, Sweden: Alfta Rehab Forlag.

Evjenth, O., and J. Hamberg. 1993. *Muscle Stretching in Manual Therapy: A Clinical Manual – The Extremities*. Alfta, Sweden: Alfta Rehab.

Magee, D. 2014. *Orthopedic Physical Assessment*. 6th ed. New York: Elsevier Saunders.

Peterson-Kendall, F., E. Kendall-McCreary, P. Geise-Provance, M. McIntyre-Rodgers, and W.A. Romani. 2005. *Muscles: Testing and Function with Posture and Pain*. 5th ed. Baltimore, Md.: Lippincott, Williams and Wilkins.

About the Authors

Paolo Sanzo is a physiotherapist at the
Victoriaville Physiotherapy Centre in
Thunder Bay, Ontario. He is an assistant
professor in the School of Kinesiology at
Lakehead University and at the Northern
Ontario School of Medicine. He is also
an instructor with the Orthopaedic
Division of the Canadian Physiotherapy
Association.

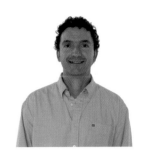

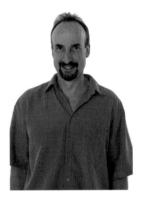

Murray MacHutchon is a physiotherapist at
Pembina Physiotherapy and Sports Injury
Clinic in Winnipeg, Manitoba. He is also an
instructor and examiner with the Orthopae-
dic Division of the Canadian Physiotherapy
Association.

The authors provide courses in the following areas:
- Length Tension Testing of the Upper and Lower Quadrants
- Muscle Energy
- Release of the Pelvic and Thoracic Outlets
- Understanding Headaches, Facial Pain and the Cranioverte-
  bral Joint Region
- Assessment and Treatment of Cervicogenic Headaches
- The Cervicothoracic Junction
- The Thoracolumbar Junction
- Sport Taping
- Neuromuscular Facilitative Taping

If you are interested in hosting a course, please do not hesitate to
contact us at www.activepotentialrehab.com.